The Ambulance

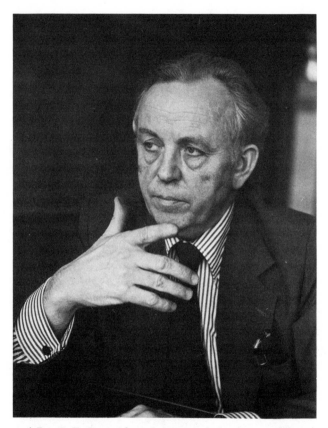

Photo of Dr. J. F. Pantridge, designer of the first mobile coronary unit and organizer of the "Flying Squad" in Belfast, Ireland, 1966. (Courtesy of Columbus Dispatch)

The Ambulance

The Story of Emergency Transportation of Sick and Wounded Through the Centuries

KATHERINE TRAVER BARKLEY

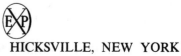

EXPOSITION PRESS   HICKSVILLE, NEW YORK

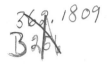

FIRST EDITION

© 1978 by Katherine T. Barkley

Library of Congress Catalog Card Number: 77-90654

ISBN 0-682-48983-2

Printed in the United States of America

To my husband, Bob, who has
helped me chase ambulances

Contents

Foreword

Dr. Warren, Professor and Chairman of the Department of Medicine at Ohio State University, received the 1976 American Heart Association's James B. Herrick award for achievement in clinical cardiology. The AHA cited Dr. Warren's teaching ability, medical leadership, and research accomplishments. Dr. Warren was the instigator of the Columbus, Ohio, program in emergency care. He was responsible for the designing of the Heartmobile and the newest Lifemobile ambulances.

There is something spine-chilling and ominous about an ambulance racing through city streets, lights flashing, and siren wailing. It signifies that something unfortunate has happened, but it also means that help is on the way. It means that somebody cares. When compared with the primitive vehicles illustrated in Mrs. Barkley's book, the modern ambulance brings an amazing array of help. Although some years ago the vehicles became more comfortable, it is remarkable that designing and equipping them as functional mini emergency units is a very recent affair. Much of this arose from an interest in mobile emergency care in the treatment of heart attack victims stemming from the original program of Dr. J. F. Pantridge in Belfast, Northern Ireland. Other lessons were learned from military experience in southeast Asia where air evacuation and emergency care became notably efficient even in hostile terrains, a far cry from the efforts of Larrey, an eighteenth century pioneer of ambulances described in this book. Fortunately we are at peace with the world today, and at home a steadily increasing number of communities are providing more and more sophisticated mobile systems of medical aid.

Interestingly enough in today's scene of improved emergency

care, the doctor usually isn't there. He has been replaced by an emergency medical technician, a paramedic, who in many ways is better able to cope with what is at the end of the run than a doctor not specifically experienced in emergency medicine. It is all part of a broad new look in emergency medical services. Hospitals have better emergency rooms, increasingly staffed by specially trained physicians, better intensive care units, and now mobile emergency care systems. They all work together. The modern ambulance system not only brings transportation to the ill and wounded, but also brings active medical care. In the case of heart attack victims who have literally dropped dead, life may be brought back. It is an important and exciting story of medical progress and Mrs. Barkley tells it well!

JAMES V. WARREN, M.D.

Preface

This pictorial history of the ambulance was initiated by Dr. Cecil Striker of Cincinnati, Ohio. He had been collecting pictures for several years and suggested that I pursue the subject. I found it to be a most fascinating study. There was a wealth of material available, but so far as I could discover, the history of the ambulance has not been written since Longmore's *Treatise on the Transport of Sick and Wounded Troops,* published in London in 1869, recorded the ambulance history of the military. I have tried to include both civilian and military ambulance history in this book.

I would like to thank all those who helped me in this compilation, and the list is very long. Much aid was also received from the National Library of Medicine and the Cincinnati, General Hospital Medical Library.

The city of Cincinnati, Ohio, has had an important part in the development of ambulances in the last century. The reader will discover this as he reads the book.

I hope the interest in this history will lead to the investigation of ambulance service in one's own community. The cooperation of every citizen is necessary. What happens when one calls an ambulance? The life you save may be your own or that of one of your family, depending on the efficiency of the ambulance system service.

A

TREATISE

ON

THE TRANSPORT OF SICK

AND

WOUNDED TROOPS.

BY

DEPUTY INSPECTOR-GENERAL T. LONGMORE, C.B.,

HONORARY SURGEON TO HER MAJESTY ;
PROFESSOR OF MILITARY SURGERY IN THE ARMY MEDICAL SCHOOL ;
CORRESPONDING MEMBER OF THE IMPERIAL SOCIETY OF SURGERY OF PARIS ;
ETC.   ETC.   ETC.

ILLUSTRATED BY NEARLY TWO HUNDRED WOOD-CUTS.

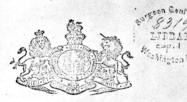

LONDON:
Printed under the Superintendence of Her Majesty's Stationery Office,
AND SOLD BY
W. CLOWES & SONS, 14, Charing Cross; HARRISON & SONS, 59, Pall Mall ;
W. H. ALLEN & Co., 13, Waterloo Place ; W. MITCHELL, Charing Cross ;
LONGMAN & Co., and TRÜBNER & Co., Paternoster Row ;
ALSO BY
A. & C. BLACK, Edinburgh; D. ROBERTSON, 90, St. Vincent Street, Glasgow ;
ALEX. THOM, Abbey Street, and E. PONSONBY, Grafton Street, Dublin.

Price Five Shillings.

22014.

12

1

The Early History
of the Ambulance

The transportation of sick and wounded has been a matter of concern through the space of history. Records of forced transport of people with leprosy or psychiatric problems can be found in ancient times. Probably the organized removal of leprosy victims from their homes was one of the first medical transport systems. The authorities were responsible for taking lepers to places where they would be isolated from the rest of the community—a measure taken to prevent the spread of the disease. The leprosy patient was often pronounced dead before he could be taken into a leprosarium; which was more a prison where he suffered punishment from heaven than a place for treatment. Patients with venereal diseases were treated in the same manner.

Many different modes of carrying have been devised. In the earliest times, no doubt, the patient was carried between two friends in whatever way was most convenient to the transporters. If there was only one person to move the invalid, the carrier's back was put to use.

Probably the next mode of carrying the sick or wounded was the use of two poles with a hammock strung between them. This type of stretcher certainly has been used for many, many years. The poles are placed on the shoulders or held at arms length by the porters.

The first wagon for transporting invalids was probably constructed about 900 A.D. The Anglo-Saxon hammock was braked by attendants who held snubbing chains around the wheels to keep the wagon from careening downhill. Even so, the person riding in the hammock must have had a rough ride swinging back and forth.

Few changes were made in the next 160 years, until the Normans came to England with a horse litter for transporting their invalids. Some adaptation of the horse litter was used until the seventeenth century. The Normans suspended a bed on poles which extended to special horse-harnesses at each end. There was a certain amount of spring in this type of litter, but the bounce must have been fatal to many a patient.

"The term ambulance," according to Henry Alan Skinner's the *Origin of Medical Terms,* "is most commonly applied to a wagon or truck in which sick and wounded are transported. In military organization the term 'field ambulance' refers to a mobile

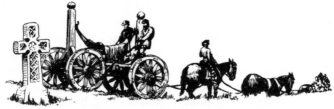

Anglo-Saxon hammock-wagon, about 900 A.D.

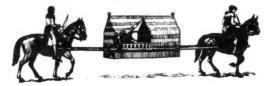

Norman horse-litter, about 1100.

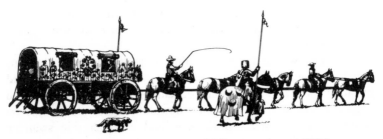

English long wagon, or whirlicote, about 1300.
(Courtesy of National Library of Medicine, Bethesda, Maryland)

unit which is equipped for the transport and emergency treatment of casualties. Such 'field hospitals' (ambulances) were introduced by Queen Isabella of Spain at the siege of Malaga in 1487 and were revived by her grandson, Charles V, at the siege of Metz in 1553."

In the late fifteenth century, Ferdinand and Isabella of Spain led their armies in a crusade against the Moors. They made the war a religious one and took it upon themselves to stay among the soldiers in order to keep up their spirits. Ferdinand shared the discomforts of the military style of life and by doing so was able to keep order. Because of his ability to lead and discipline his men, the Spanish army was considered to be one of the finest military organizations of its time. Volunteers from countries all over Europe flocked to Spain to become part of their military organization. Consequently, the Spaniards learned the art of war, especially from the Swiss mercenaries. Gonzalo de Cordoba, a Spanish captain, became familiar with the European methods and developed military tactics which made the Spaniards the finest soldiers in Europe.

New military ideas were combined with the old. Ferdinand and Isabella took an unprecedented interest in the welfare of their troops. Surgical and medical supplies were gathered together and the first military hospitals, *ambulancias,* were established as special tents for the wounded.

It was not until some three hundred years later, however, that some arrangement was made to move the wounded to the field hospitals during the battles and to bring aid to the wounded who could not be moved.

LARREY'S FLYING AMBULANCE

Dominique-Jean Larrey was born at Baudean, France, on July 8, 1766. He was orphaned as a child and little is known of his childhood. He did eventually study under his uncle, Alexis, who had founded a special school of surgery in Toulouse.

He completed his studies in Toulouse and decided to visit other universities in order to acquire as much knowledge as possible in his chosen profession.

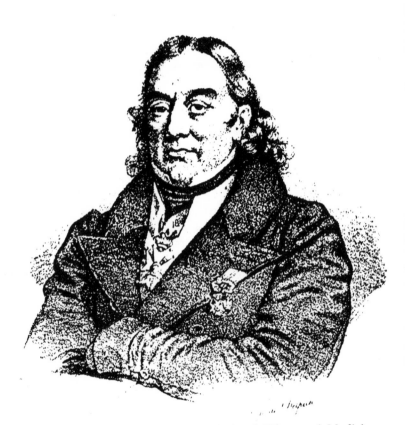

A portrait of Larrey. (Courtesy of National Library of Medicine, Bethesda, Maryland)

When he arrived in Paris he learned that there were vacancies in the navy for assistant surgeons, so he applied and was accepted. He travelled on foot for the 350 miles to Brest where he was to embark. Here he spent several months learning everything he could about ships and the sea and all medical and surgical equipment for which he was responsible.

The ship finally sailed in early May and Larrey was seasick for most of the voyage. He described his illness and all the treatments he tried in a published paper. They landed at Belle Isle, an island north of Newfoundland, which was French territory.

In his writing Larrey described in great detail how he treated the large number of cases of scurvy and other ailments which the crew suffered.

When he arrived back in Paris during the winter of 1789, the signs of the coming revolution were beginning to be evident. Larrey was studying clinical surgery under M. Desault when large numbers of wounded civilians were brought in to the Hotel Dieu. The wounded had been in a crowd that was demonstrating against the owners of a paper factory. The owners of the factory called in the Swiss guard with artillery. Many more riots followed and the fall of the Bastile brought more and more wounded to the hospital. Larrey had an excellent chance to study the type of wounds which were received in battle. As a result of this experience Larrey developed a semi-circular surgical needle which had a lancet-shaped cutting point and an eye grooved to hold the suture. The Royal Academy of Surgery presented him with a gold medal for this contribution to the surgical practice.

In 1792 the Prussians and Austrians declared "war against kings, and peace with all peoples." The French armies were not prepared to fight off the attackers and they dropped their weapons and ran. Larrey was ordered to join the Army of the Rhine under Marshall Luchner. For several weeks, the medical personnel prepared dressings and discussed military surgery.

There was a battle between the French, under Marshall Custine—who had replaced Marshall Luchner—and the Prussians at Spires. Here Larrey had his first experience of a serious military engagement. Ambulances were required to be stationed about two and a half miles in the rear of the army. Wounded were left on the battlefield until the fight was over when the ambulances went to pick them up and take them to field hospitals.

Larrey was distressed that the wounded were neglected for so long a period of time and that most of them died before they reached the hospital. It was this situation which led him to try to develop a new ambulance system which would bring help to the wounded and also carry them away from the danger of the battlefield.

After several battles Larrey's shock at the lack of immediate care for the wounded caused him to approach the Commissary-General Villemansy with the idea of special mobile ambulances. He was given authority to develop his plans.

At first, Larrey thought of moving the wounded on pack-horses with litters strapped on the horses' backs. However, he decided in favor of light carriages.

Larrey saw his ambulance wagons used in the mountains near Konigstein in Prussia. The terrible experience of seeing the battle at such close quarters was offset by the realization that his ambulances were saving so many lives.

Young Napoleon Bonaparte, in a short and successful campaign, had driven the Austrians out of Northern Italy, and while enjoying his new military prominence, he put his efforts into improving the equipment of his armies. He was impressed with the reputation of Larrey whose humane treatment of the battle wounded appealed to Napoleon. Larrey was ordered to join the Army of Italy and organize ambulance service similar to the one he had initiated in 1793 for the Army of the Rhine.

Before Larrey's innovation in ambulance service, the army regulations required the ambulance-wagons to be stationed to the rear of the armies. The wagons were heavy and clumsy, primarily used for transporting surgeons and equipment. Baron Percy, Larrey's senior partner who shared with him the responsibility for the surgery department of the army, designed a wagon on four wheels with a pole down the center, making a kind of saddle which the surgeons straddled while riding to the wounded after the battle was over.

Larrey designed a lightweight, two-wheeled ambulance which stayed with the troops and allowed the surgeons to work on the battlefield. He also used these wagons to pick up wounded and transport them out to hospitals. These were called "flying ambulances" because they stayed with the "flying artillery" on the battlefield.

Larrey directed the ambulance service during Napoleon's Italian campaign of 1797, and in 1798 he organized the health service for the army in Egypt. It was here that he used pack animals for transporting the wounded, even devising a litter which could be strapped on the back of a camel.

He founded a medical school in Milan, Italy. Larrey became surgeon of the French Imperial Guard in 1801. He served in some twenty-six campaigns in the Napoleonic Wars from 1805 to Waterloo in 1815.

While performing over two hundred amputations in the bitter cold of Borodino, Russia, Larrey discovered the value of freezing in amputations.

Larrey had many other firsts to his credit. He was responsible for the first two successful amputations of the leg at the hip joint in 1803. A method of disarticulating the humerus at the shoulder joint is called Larrey's Amputation. He discovered that maggots were good for clearing up infection and that trachoma was contagious. He encouraged leg fracture patients to get out of bed as soon as possible; and he was probably the first to recognize that granular conjunctivitis was contagious.

Larrey's son, Baron Felix-Hippolyte Larrey (1808-1895), was chief surgeon of the Army Medical Corps and a pioneer in the use of ether.

It is interesting to note that the same pictures of pack animals used for transporting wounded have appeared in military medical manuals from the time of Larrey's design for their use until modern times in the Vietnam War.

Ambulance wagons were modified and adapted both for civilian and military use, but few major changes were made for the next one hundred years until the motor ambulance came into common use in the early 1900s.

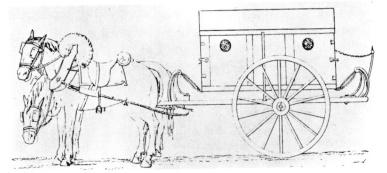

Larrey's light ambulance that was in use during the Napoleonic Wars.

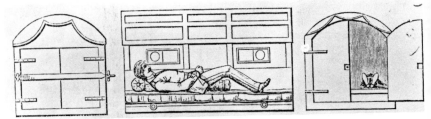

From left to right: the front, the interior, and the rear views of Larrey's flying ambulance cart.

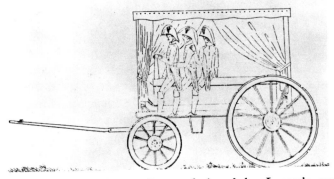

The Ambulance du Baron Percy, designed by Larrey's senior partner.

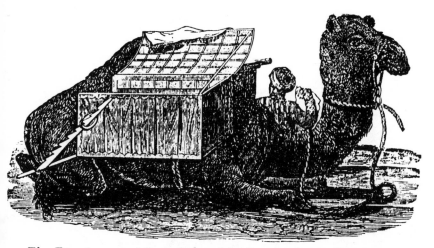

The Egyptian camel-litter designed by Larrey during Napoleon's campaign in that country. The animal is seated, and the litter shown on the one side is open, ready to receive a patient.

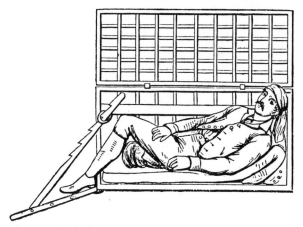

An interior view of the camel-litter. One side has been removed to show the position of a wounded man who had been placed in it after having undergone amputation above the knee.

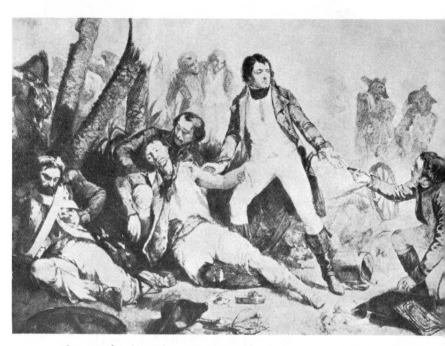

A reproduction of a painting now to be seen at Val-de-Grace, the Military Museum in Paris. It is an idealized version of Larrey proceeding with an amputation on the field of battle. (From Wangensteen, Owen H., and Wangensteen, Sarah D.: "Successful pre-Listerian Antiseptic Management of Compound Fracture: Crowther (1802), Larrey, (1824), and Bennion (ca. 1840), Surgery 69: 811-824, 1971)

CARRIAGE FOR CHOLERA PATIENTS—1832

A surgeon, George Glover, Esq., invented a carriage which he thought would be advantageous to the cholera patient. In the interior, the patient would lie on a movable couch, which was kept warm by a mattress of heated salt. The salt was kept heated at each of the station houses, by means of a sand-bath. When the signal was given, the hot salt was put into the mattress and covered with blankets, and the carriage was immediately driven off to get the patient.

According to J. Knapp, in a letter to the editor of the *London Medical Gazette* dated 1832, the advantages of such a conveyance were: "The curative process commences the instant the patient is put into the carriage; time is saved which can be given to the care of the patient; the patient may be driven to the hospital so speedily that the hospitals may be less numerous and located at greater distances from each other, and removed from a crowded part of the town to a more wholesome locality so that the medical attendants will be less exposed to contagion."

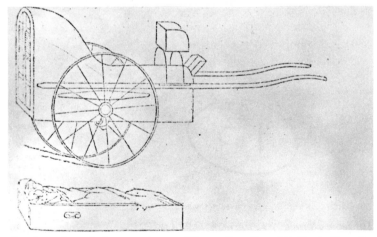

Carriage for cholera patients. (From London Medical Gazette, 1832.)

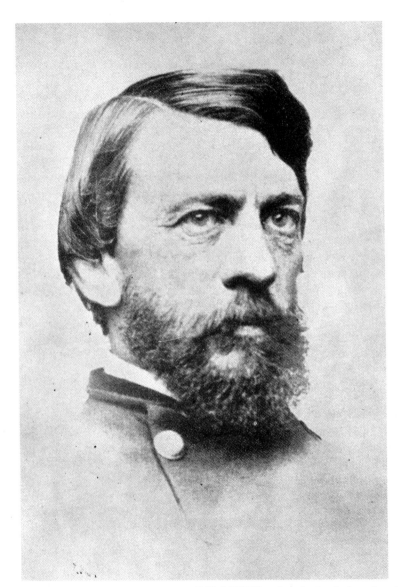

Surgeon Jonathan Letterman (1824-1872) who devised the plan of field hospitalization and evacuation that has influenced that service in every modern army. (Courtesy of the Armed Forces Institute of Pathology)

2

Ambulances During
the American Civil War

Although ambulance service was suggested to the army in 1861, nothing was done about it. However, on June 13, 1861, Lincoln approved an order creating the United States Sanitary Commission. The Reverend Henry Bellows, a Unitarian minister, was president of the Commission which became the Red Cross of the Civil War. Hospital transports were maintained and directed by the Sanitary Commission.

The two Bull Run engagements were disastrous for the Union. Ambulances were too few, too far between, and too late, driven by civilian drunkards and thieves who ran when they heard the guns. The Quartermaster Corps decided to use two-wheeled ambulances thinking they would ride better. Not a few men were jarred to death, and the wagon became known as the "avalanche." Fortunately, these were abandoned after the first year of the war. Most of them had broken down and were beyond repair at that time.

Jonathan Letterman (1824-1872) organized the field medical service of the Union Army. He was the son of a physician, Jonathan Letterman, Sr. The younger Jonathan received his medical education at Jefferson Medical College, Philadelphia, receiving the M.D. degree in 1849. Immediately following graduation he passed the examination by the U.S. Army examining board in New York and was appointed assistant surgeon.

For twelve years, Letterman was located in the western and southwestern frontiers and was involved in wars with the Indians. The experience he received in improvising treatment, and transporting the wounded under the difficult conditions of such warfare, was excellent training for later responsibilities during the Civil War.

At the outbreak of the war in 1861, Letterman was assigned to duty with the Army of the Potomac. In 1862 he was promoted to major and surgeon and was appointed medical director of that army under the command of Major General McClellan. In this position, he completely reorganized the field medical service, creating an effective mobile hospital organization and provided ambulance service for the evacuation of battle casualties.

The organization was effective at Chancellorsville, Antietam, and Gettysburg and was then adapted for use throughout the Union army. In fact, the Letterman basic plan of field hospitalization and evacuation has influenced the medical service in all succeeding wars. In 1911, the War Department designated a hospital in San Francisco the Letterman General Hospital, in honor of the man who revolutionized the system of care of the wounded on the battlefield.

In 1864, an act was brought before the U.S. Congress by the War Department. The law was finally passed that definitely established a uniform army ambulance plan. The act was entitled "An Act to Establish a Uniform System of Ambulances in the Armies of the United States."

One of the features of the new act was that it separated the Ambulance Transport from all other transport services of the army. The whole of the ambulance service, personnel, vehicles, and administration was to be the responsibility of the head of the medical department of the army who was to establish an ambulance corps. The act spelled out who was responsible for each phase of the ambulance system and declared that the personnel should wear special uniforms and the wagons should be specially marked.

1861—THE TWO-WHEELED FINLEY

Every regiment in the early part of the Civil War possessed one or two two-wheeled ambulances, such as the Finley wagon.

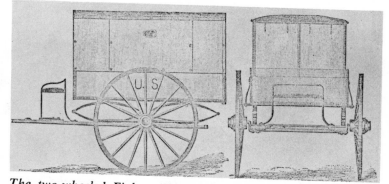

The two-wheeled Finley. (Medical and Surgical History of the War of Rebellion—1861 to 1865, published in 1866)

The two-wheelers proved unsuccessful in their use. They were too light and unsuited to the rough roads of the country and easily broken. They accommodated only two or three patients.

THE "RUCKER" AMBULANCE

The Rucker ambulance wagon was constructed under the direction of Major General Rucker of the United States Quartermaster's Department. It was recommended for adoption as the regulation ambulance wagon of the United States Army. It acommodated both ambulatory and recumbent patients (four recumbent or eight to ten ambulatory patients).

The Rucker wagon, in a modified form, gained one of the prizes offered for the best kind of ambulance wagon at the Paris Exposition in 1867. Dr. Thomas Evans of Paris was the modifier, giving more elasticity to the stretchers, adding extra springs to the floor, and improving ventilation. Dr. Evans also added seats for attendants at the rear of the wagon.

During the Civil War Rucker ambulance "trains" were a common sight.

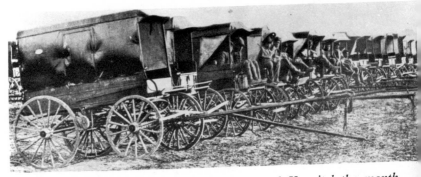

An ambulance train "parked" at Harewood Hospital the month Gettysburg was fought.

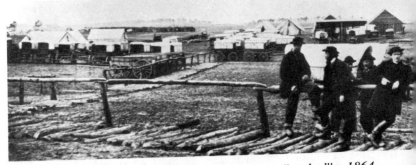

Ambulances and medical supply wagons "parked"—1864.

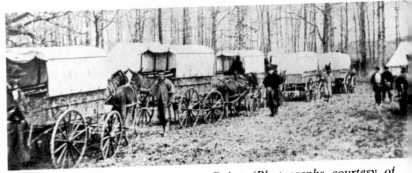

A train of ambulances at City Point. (Photographs courtesy of the National Library of Medicine, Bethesda, Maryland)

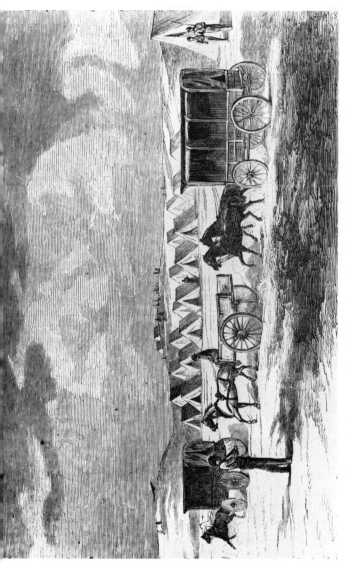

An ambulance train during the Charlestown Harbor campaign coming from the trenches with wounded. (Wood engraving from Harper's Weekly, vol. 7, September 12, 1863. Courtesy of National Library of Medicine, Bethesda, Maryland)

STEAMBOAT HOSPITALS

In 1862, Fort Donelson fell to Union forces. Severe injuries were treated on the spot. Others went to the rear of the fighting via ambulance where they stayed until further arrangements were made. Usually the next move was by steamer down the Cumberland River to hospitals along the Ohio River.

The Cincinnati Branch of the U.S. Sanitary Commission chartered the steamboat *Allen Collier,* a 133-ton stern-wheel vessel built in Cincinnati. The ship was stocked with hospital supplies and staffed with surgeons and nurses. There was such confusion and resentment on the part of the state equipped transports that the hospital ship almost returned home from Fort Donelson without any passengers. However, the staff insisted on helping the wounded and managed to take eighty-one men to a military hospital in Cincinnati. This was the first recorded trip of a United States Sanitary Commission hospital steamer in the West.

Many other boats were used for transporting the wounded to hospitals. Unfortunately, military officers were not responsible to a private system of transports and therefore did not have to obey orders which came from the volunteers serving on the ships. Eventually the United States government took over the Sanitary Commission's boats including the doctors and male nurses.

The Fanny Bullitt—*1862*

The steamer *Fanny Bullitt* was a side-wheeler of good dimensions and fair speed of which J. A. Lemcke became commander and five-sixths owner in 1861. Lemcke, a Union sympathizer and in charge of the steamer, wanted to offer the *Fanny's* services to the Union Forces. The Kentucky owner, a Southerner, would not let the boat be used against the South. Lemcke determined to buy the boat, which he did with the help of a friend.

Without the authority of the War Department, Lemcke enrolled himself as a captain of "horse marines" and attached his boat to an Illinois regiment at Shawneetown on the Wabash River. He and his crew thought they were being highly patriotic in helping to bring the Union victory.

Early in 1862, when the Federal forces had established military posts at Paducah and Smithland, General Grant ordered Lemcke to report in Cairo with the *Fanny Bullitt*. On their arrival, the boat was ordered to anchor in the middle of the Ohio River and await orders.

Fort Donelson on the Cumberland River surrendered on February 13, 1862. The *Fanny Bullitt* was ordered to load up and take away the first of the wounded men from the battlefield to unknown hospitals. The battlefield was knee-deep in wet yellow clay which made it very difficult to get the wounded aboard ship. The Cumberland River was high and rushing with flood waters. Surgeons were needed on the battlefield so Lemcke left without a single doctor or nurse on board. There were two hundred wounded and their destination was left entirely to the captain's judgment. To add to the problem, the pilot, Barney Seals, was extremely drunk. Captain Lemcke visualized the two hundred suffering passengers shipwrecked and drowning, to add to their already deplorable state.

A woman, Mrs. Bickerdyke, had somehow come aboard and was washing and binding up the soldiers' wounds. She was a volunteer and the only woman on the boat. She took charge and the crew were so grateful they followed her every command.

There was no hospital at Paducah that could take his passengers. They went four hundred miles further to Louisville without Mother Bickerdyke. She stayed in Cairo where she was also needed desperately.

At Shawneetown, Illinois, men were taken ashore by local volunteers. At Henderson, Kentucky, the Kentucky wounded were taken in. At Evansville, the Indiana men were looked after by the charitable citizens of that town.

Governor Morton of Indianapolis ordered supplies, doctors, and nurses to accompany the remaining patients to Louisville. Here there were hospital accommodations, but because of the flooding

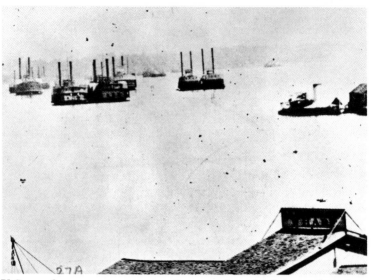

U.S. gunboats, transports, and a monitor (right), anchored at Cairo, Illinois during the Civil War. The sign on the wharfboat in the foreground says: U.S. QUARTERMASTER'S WHARF. None of the boats are identified, but the Fanny Bullitt very well may be one of the side-wheelers in the distance at the left. (Courtesy of S. & D. Reflector *published by Sons and Daughters of Pioneer Rivermen)*

river the boat sailed right into Forty-eighth Street among the stores of the city in order to unload the patients into spring-wagon ambulances.

Captain Lemcke first published this story in the *Indiana Magazine of History,* 1905, under the title "Reminiscences of an Indianian."

Jacob Strader—*1863 to 1864*

The *Jacob Strader* was the largest inland river craft ever built to date, measuring some 357 feet in length. As indicated by the picture, she was a side-wheeler and was powered by low pressure

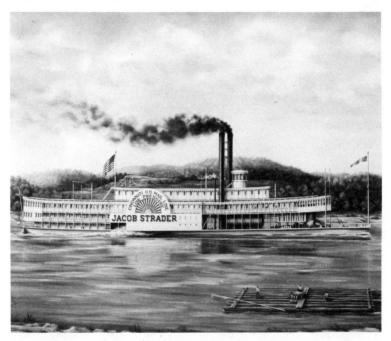

The Jacob Strader, a mail boat used to transport the wounded to hospitals in Cincinnati during the war. (Courtesy of John J. Strader)

steam engines. The boat was all glassed in and boasted a round pilot house, situated just ahead of the stacks.

Built by Jacob Strader at the Old East End Shipyards in Cincinnati in 1853, its primary function was to carry the U.S. mail (just in front of the boiler). The *Strader* plied a course between Pittsburgh and New Orleans. She carried passengers in a luxurious manner during peacetime. At the time of the Civil War, she transported troops and brought wounded soldiers to the hospital in Cincinnati.

3

Geneva Convention
of 1864

Jean Henri Dunant (1828-1910) had two inspirations to set about forming the humanitarian movement we know today as the Red Cross—Florence Nightingale's service in the Crimean War (1854-56) and his own experience on the battlefield of Solferino in 1859.

French and Italian troops under the command of Napoleon, numbering 138,000 men, stormed the heights above the plains of Lombardy held by 129,000 Austrians under Emperor Francis Joseph.

Wounded and dying were brought into nearby villages. Most of them gathered in Castiglione, where they occupied every available space in the town. Here Dunant established an emergency hospital in an old church and did what he could to relieve the suffering. A number of women volunteered to help with the pitifully inadequate supplies to minister impartially to the victims of both sides.

Dunant strongly promoted more humane and more extensive aid to wounded soldiers in times of battle. He lectured on his experiences and made a plea for some organization of people interested in furthering this cause.

M. Gustav Moynier, president of one society where Dunant lectured, and a man of independent wealth, became very much interested. Dr. Louis Appia, a physician and philanthropist, and Adolph Ador, a counsellor in Geneva, also took up the cause.

These men were able to enlist the cooperation of Dufour, the general of the Swiss Army, and together they called a meeting of the "Society of Public Utility" of Geneva to consider a "proposition relative to the formation of permanent societies for the relief of wounded soldiers." The meeting took place in February, 1863. As a result, a committee was appointed with M. Moynier as chairman to examine methods of organizing a plan.

M. Moynier and his committee decided to call together men from many countries who sympathized with their ideas. Beginning the following October 26, the sessions went on for four days and resulted in the calling of an international convention to be held the following year, 1864, in Geneva.

The Geneva Treaty was adopted and a permanent international committee based in Geneva was formed. One of the first actions necessary was the securing of agreements of some important European countries to recognize the neutrality of hospitals, of the sick and wounded, of all persons connected with relief service, and the adoption of a protective sign or badge.

The Swiss Federal Council and the Emperor of France were the first to sign the treaty, soon to be followed by ten other governments. They agreed that the badge should be a red cross on a white background, worn on the arm by all persons in the act of aiding the sick and wounded.

The treaty also provided for the neutrality of all sanitary supplies, ambulances, surgeons, nurses, attendants, and the sick and wounded, and for their safe conduct when the red-cross-sign was in view.

The sign of the red cross was chosen as a compliment to the Swiss republic who had initiated the whole activity through Henri Dunant and the central committee. The Swiss flag is a white cross on a red background, and the Red Cross badge chosen was these colors in reverse.

Although the Geneva Convention which originated the Red Cross organization was international, the Societies in each nation are independent, each one governing itself according to the national needs.

The function of the International Committee in Geneva, determined by the 1864 conference, is to serve as an intermediate agent between National Committees and facilitate their communications with each other.

The National Committees are charged with the direction of the work in their own countries.

Following are the Articles of the Geneva Convention:

ARTICLES OF THE
INTERNATIONAL RED CROSS TREATY
CONVENTION OF GENEVA FOR THE
AMELIORIZATION OF THE CONDITIONS OF THE
WOUNDED IN ARMIES AT THE FIELD
AUGUST *22, 1864*

ARTICLE 1: Ambulances and military hospitals shall be acknowledged to be neuter, and as such shall be protected and respected by belligerents as long as any sick or wounded may be therein.

Such neutrality shall cease if the ambulances or hospitals should be held by a military force.

ARTICLE 2. Persons employed in hospitals and ambulances, comprising the staff for superintendence, medical service, administration, transport of wounded, as well as chaplains, shall participate in the benefit of neutrality while so employed and so long as there remain any wounded to bring in or to succor.

ARTICLE 3: The persons designated in the preceding Article may, even after occupation by the enemy, continue to fulfill their duties in the hospital or ambulance which they serve or may withdraw in order to rejoin the corps to which they belong.

Under such circumstances, when those persons shall cease from their functions, they shall be delivered by the occupying army to the outposts of the enemy.

ARTICLE 4: As the equipment of military hospitals remains subject to the laws of war, persons attached to such hospitals cannot, in withdrawing, carry away any articles but such as are their private property. Under the same circumstances an ambulance shall, on the contrary, retain its equipment.

ARTICLE 5: Inhabitants of the country who may bring help to the wounded shall be respected and shall remain free. The generals of the belligerent powers shall make it their care to inform the inhabitants of the appeal addressed to their humanity, and of the neutrality which will be the consequence of it.

Any wounded man entertained and taken care of in a house shall be considered as a protection thereto. Any inhabitant who shall have entertained wounded men in his house shall be exempted from the quartering of troops, as well as from a part of the contributions of war which may be imposed.

ARTICLE 6: Wounded or sick soldiers shall be entertained and taken care of, to whatever nation they may belong.

Commanders-in-chief shall have the power to deliver immediately to the outposts of the enemy soldiers who have been wounded in an engagement, when circumstances permit this to be done, and with the consent of both parties.

Those who are recognized, after they are healed, as incapable of serving, shall be sent back to their country.

The others may also be sent back on condition of not again bearing arms during continuance of the war.

Evacuations, together with the person under whose directions they take place, shall be protected by an absolute neutrality.

ARTICLE 7: A distinctive and uniform flag shall be adopted for hospitals, ambulances, and evacuations. It must, on every occasion, be accompanied by the national flag. An arm-badge (brassard) shall also be allowed for individuals neutralized, but the delivery thereof shall be left to military authority.

The flag and arm-badge shall bear a red cross on a white ground.

ARTICLE 8: The details of execution of the present convention shall be regulated by the commanders-in-chief of belligerent armies, according to the instructions of their respective governments, and in conformity with the general principles laid down in this convention.

This event in 1864 changed the whole inhumane practice of leaving wounded on the battlefield, and led to the development of humanitarian programs throughout the world for serving people's needs in peacetime and wartime.

AMERICAN RED CROSS

While Dunant was organizing relief societies in Europe a similar organization was functioning in the American Civil War under the United States Sanitary Commission 1861-66. Dr. Henry W. Bellows, a New York clergyman, was the leader of this effort along with nearly one hundred women in New York City.

The purpose of the Sanitary Commission was to carry out a program of relief services for soldiers on the battlefield. Charles S. P. Bowles represented this commission at the 1864 Geneva Convention as an unofficial delegate from the United States. Bowles was able to cite many experiences which helped the Geneva Convention to formulate policies. Many people were concerned that volunteers on the battlefield would hamper military operations. Bowles said this was not a problem, according to their experience in the Civil War.

The Sanitary Commission preceded the American Red Cross by some twenty years. After the Civil War many attempts were made to form an American Red Cross and to influence the United States government to sign the agreement of the Geneva Convention. All efforts failed until Clara Barton came on the scene. Miss Barton was a volunteer worker among the wounded during the Civil War, although she worked independently of the Commission.

During a trip to Europe after the War, Clara Barton became acquainted with the Red Cross organization. She worked with the Red Cross during the Franco-Prussian War, then returned home to found an American Red Cross and to persuade President James Garfield to recommend to the Congress their support of the Geneva Convention. Garfield was assassinated shortly after he agreed to carry the cause to Congress, but President Chester Arthur carried out his predecessor's promise. The Senate ratified the Geneva Convention in 1882.

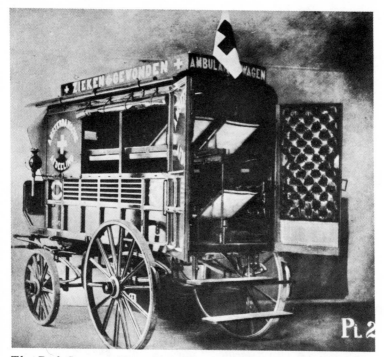

The Red Cross emblem displayed on a Dutch ambulance wagon. (Courtesy of National Library of Medicine, Bethesda, Maryland)

The American Society immediately began to prepare for disaster relief during peacetime. In this effort, the Society was different than in most other countries where the Red Cross became active only during wartime. However, in 1884 The American Red Cross introduced an amendment to the International Red Cross which led to the reorganization of all national groups for disaster relief as well as war service.

The first wartime service came in the Spanish-American War of 1898.

4

"A Treatise on
the Transport of Sick
and Wounded Troops—1869"

BY

DEPUTY INSPECTOR-GENERAL T. LONGMORE, C.B.

T. Longmore was Honorary Surgeon to Her Majesty, Queen Victoria. He was professor of Military Surgery in the Army Medical School and a Corresponding Member of the Imperial Society of Surgery of Paris. His *Treatise* was printed under the Superintendence of Her Majesty's Stationary Office in London in 1869. The dedication in the book was worded as follows:

> *To His Esteemed Colleagues at Netley*
> *To Whose Affectionate Care He Is So*
> *Greatly Indebted*
> *For Recovery from Recent Severe Illness,*
> *This Attempt*
> *To Prepare the Way for Further Improvements*
> *In the Means*
> *Of Aiding Wounded Soldiers in the*
> *Time of War,*
> *Is Dedicated by the Author,*
> *As a Mark*
> *Of His Sincere Regard and Gratitude*

In the introduction of his book, Longmore comments on the fact that the medical and surgical departments of military organizations are the most defective. This was true all over the

40

world wherever armies existed. Also, it was generally agreed that the ambulance systems were the least satisfactory sections of the medical and surgical divisions.

Longmore discovered that up to that time no systematic work had been published on the subject of ambulance systems in any language. He felt the need for a "practical work of reference in which could be found an account of what had been done in the past, an explanation of existing arrangements, and such guiding principles as may not only serve the purpose of preventing a repetition of former failures, but also of steering the way to future improvements." This is the information which Longmore furnished in his *Treatise*.

In 1854, the Director-General of the British Army Medical Department, knowing there would be many defects in the ambulance carts and wagons sent to Turkey with the army, asked for medical officers to make suggestions for their improvement. There were only a few responses. The whole subject was so new to most of the officers, they had little constructive criticism to offer.

During the Crimean War, many people suggested better ways of transporting sick and wounded but most of the suggested improvements were totally impractical for the particular geographic locations in which they were to be used.

In 1867, the Universal Exhibition at Paris gave a fresh stimulus to the study of ambulance transport. A committee of persons from the "Societies for Help to Wounded in Time of War" of different countries brought to the Exhibition a large collection of ambulance wagons which had been used in the past or had been designed for future use. Prizes were offered for the best forms of hand litters, wheeled litters, and wagons.

Several governments exhibited the authorized ambulance of their countries. Longmore was fortunate to have seen and tested the conveyances at the Exhibition. This opportunity enabled him to gather much of the material for his *Treatise*.

As for the British Ambulance Service, Longmore says it was necessary to study each of the colonial possessions of Great Britain in order to find the right vehicle for the particular terrain.

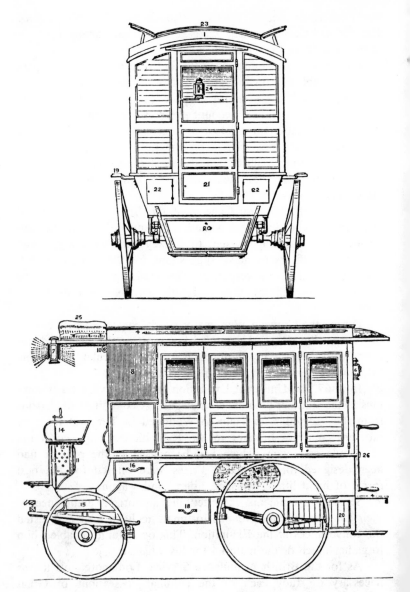

Side and rear views of the Locati sick-transport wagon.

His book is very detailed, including many specifications for the conveyances described.

Opposite are some illustrations found in the book.

FIELD TRANSPORTS

Director General Smith's Sick-Transport Wagon was used in the Crimean War but was found to be too heavy, especially when the horses were deficient in strength, the drivers untrained, and the roads bad. The weight of the wagon was twenty-two hundred pounds when empty. Add to this the weight of ten patients, two drivers, and all their gear. The distance between the front and back wheels contributed to the difficulty in handling. Although the four rear compartments were ventilated, the soldiers felt restrained and helpless because they could not sit up in the narrow compartments.

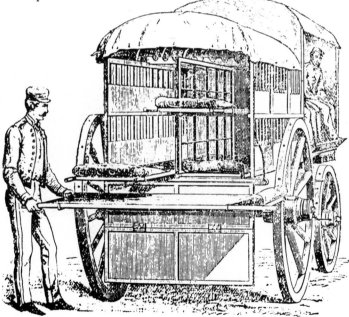

General Smith's sick-transport wagon.

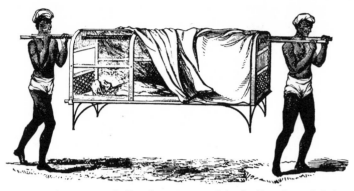

Dr. Francis' improved dhooley was used in India. One deficiency in this conveyance was in its weight (with a patient) which would be difficult for shoulder-carrying over rough ground for any long period of time.

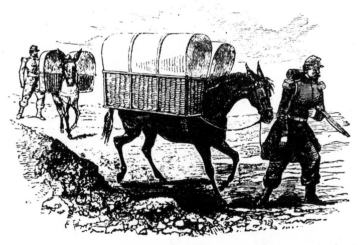

Mule-panniers are long wicker baskets in the form of cradles covered by canopies of canvas supported on four hoops. They would only be used when all other regular litters are in use. They cannot be folded up, but would be useful for those soldiers too weak to walk.

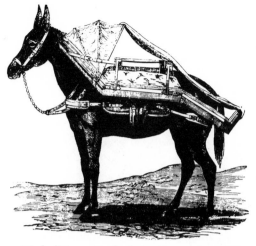

Mule-litter attached to its pack saddle.

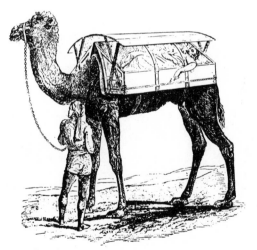

Brett's camel dhooley was attached to the animal by straps of strong ropes threaded through iron rings and placed over the saddle. If needed, curtains could be hung from the roof of the litter.

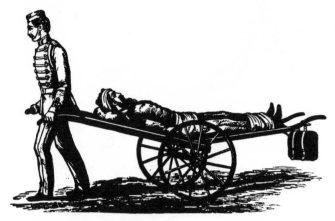

Gablenz's wheeled litter offered the patient a secure position. The stretcher is light and easily separated from wheels when necessary.

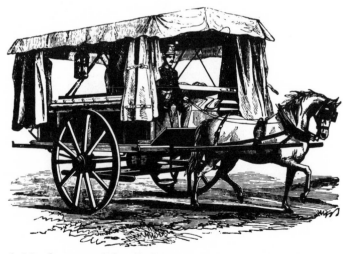

Guthrie's flat-topped hospital conveyance cart was designed for carrying two patients lying on spring stretchers on the floor and a third in a stretcher slung from the roof. There was room for nine people sitting on seats.

The British ambulance wagon was built with separate compartments for the recumbent and sitting patients. Two moveable stretchers occupied the central portion of the floor. Seats were for those who could sit up. Later it was decided that it was not advantageous to have patients both sitting up and lying down in the same area. Two horses were used to draw the wagon. A canvas cover was supported by moveable hoops. A wicker basket was suspended from the roof to hold knapsacks. Firearms had a special compartment.

This wagon gave good service in England but was not satisfactory when used abroad, probably due to the weight of the wagon and the bad roads.

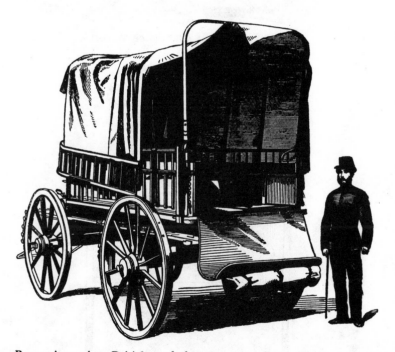

Rear view of a British ambulance wagon from Thomas Longmore's Treatise on the Transport of Sick and Wounded Troops. *(Courtesy of National Library of Medicine, Bethesda, Maryland)*

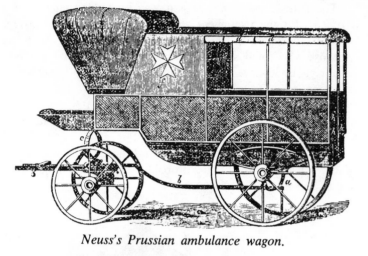

Neuss's Prussian ambulance wagon.

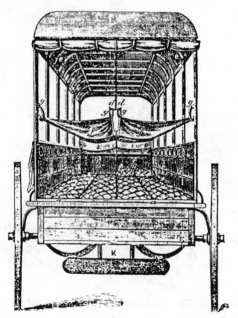

Perspective view of the interior of the Evans Sick Transport Wagon.

The Wheeling Rosecrans Wagon (1864), along with the Rucker, was extensively used during the latter part of the Civil War in the United States. It was first constructed in Wheeling, Virginia, according to the designs of General Rosecrans. It was light enough to be drawn by two horses and carried both sitting and recumbent patients, ten or twelve sitting or two or three lying down.

The principal feature of this wagon was the fact that the seats could be converted into litters. Under the driver's seat there was a box which contained equipment for field use. A five-gallon water tank was secured to the back of the carriage.

This wagon was considered to be too high from the ground for handling recumbent patients. It was also a very bumpy riding vehicle.

THE USE OF RAILWAYS TO
TRANSPORT THE SICK AND WOUNDED

A chapter on the "Use of Railways as regards to transportation of sick and wounded in Time of War" is the last one in Longmore's *Treatise*. He enumerates the advantages of Railway transportation:

1. Important strategical advantage of relief of the active part of an army from the encumbrance of sick and disabled men.
2. Advantage of rapid conveyance of ineffective soldiers in vehicles secure against attack where best hospital service is available for most quickly restoring them to active service.
3. The ability of the railway to disperse wounded and sick among many facilities contributes to better care for each one.
4. The use of railways for transportation of wounded to hospital reduces the amount of ambulance equipment and field hospital organizations needed to accompany each army.

Railways were used in the Italian campaign of 1859, the German-Danish war of 1864, the Civil War in the United States, and the war between Prussia and Austria in 1866. Each of these

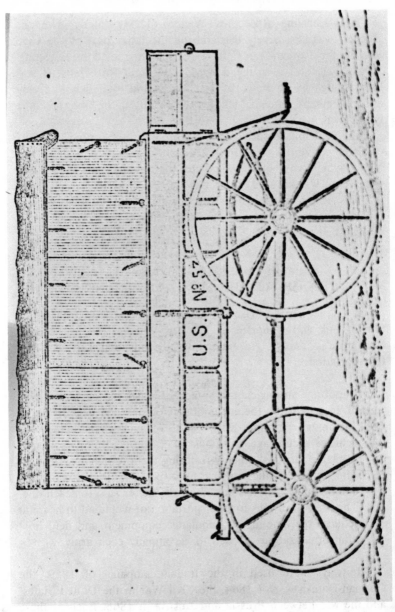

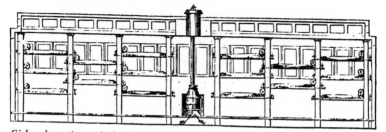

Side elevation of the interior of an American hospital railway car.

campaigns was described by Longmore to show the advantages of the use of railways for transporting sick and wounded.

Transportation of the Wounded by Railway of the Army of the Potomac, June 1863

Longmore in his *Treatise* quotes from *Medical Recollections of the Army of the Potomac* by J. Letterman, M.D., New York, 1866, to show how the wounded were transported during the Civil War. He prefaces the extract by saying, "Dr. Letterman's work is not much known in this country and the following extract, describing the arrangements for transporting a large number of patients by railway on the army leaving Fredericksburg to Aquia Creek depot in June 1863, will be of interest:

The railroad from Fredericksburg to Aquia Creek depot had a single track with short sidings. Over this road had to be transported, in a very short time, more than nine thousand wounded and sick, with all the hospital tents, medical and surgical supplies, stores, etc., required for their care, together with the accumulated supplies of the Quartermaster's Commissary and Ordinance Departments. I sent Medical Inspector Taylor to Aquia Creek to receive the wounded and send them by hospital ships to Washington. The network of telegraph wires made by the Signal Corps enabled me to regulate the shipment of this large number of men without difficulty or accident. I had directed that all who could not sit up, or would

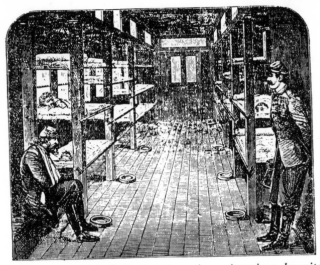

Perspective view of half the interior of an American hospital car conveying wounded soldiers.

be injured by so doing, should be carried by hand upon the beds they occupied in the hospital (some of which were more than a mile from the railway), the beds placed upon hay in the cars, removed carefully from the train and placed in the transports, so that the sufferers should not be removed from the beds on which they lay in the camp hospitals until they reached the hospitals in Washington. Medical officers, with supplies, accompanied every train, and when required, were sent with their men to Washington. Many of those most severely wounded, cases in which the femur was extensively fractured, assured me they had not suffered the slightest discomfort or fatigue up to the time of their being placed on the transports.

The removal of this convoy of sick and wounded numbering nine thousand and twenty-five, began on the morning of the twelfth of June, and before six o'clock in the evening of the fourteenth of June, all had left the depot at Aquia for Washington."

5

A Report to the Surgeon General on the Transport of Sick and Wounded by Pack Animals

George A. Otis,
Assistant Surgeon, U.S. Army, 1877

Dr. George Alexander Otis, born in 1830 in Boston, Massachusetts, was graduated from Princeton with a B.A. in 1850 and an M.A. in the Medical Department of the University of Pennsylvania in 1851. He was in private practice in Springfield, Massachusetts, at the beginning of the Civil War and was appointed surgeon of the twenty-eighth Massachusetts Volunteers.

In 1864, he was assigned to the Surgeon General's office as assistant to the curator, then curator of the Army Medical Museum primarily concerned with gathering data for a surgical history of the Civil War. His most noteworthy accomplishment was the three surgical volumes of the *Medical and Surgical History of the War of the Rebellion.*

His Circular No. 9, "Report to the Surgeon General on the Transport of Sick and Wounded by Pack Animals," published in 1877 has a modern parallel in pages 80 and 81 of Army Field Manual 8-35 "Transportation of the Sick and Wounded," 1970. Photographs on these pages show wounded being moved in this fashion in the Vietnam War.

Otis's main purpose in Circular 9 was to show that preparation must be made, equipment researched, and personnel drilled for rapid battlefield medical evacuation. Otis described the evacuation

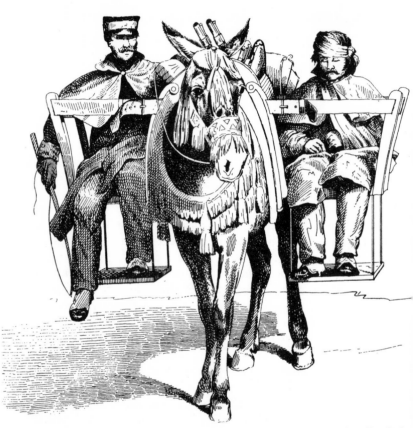

Method of transporting the wounded of the French, English, and Sardinian armies in the Crimea in 1854-55.

of fifty-nine wounded from the Battle of the Little Big Horn by travois over thirty rugged miles without "accident or personal inconvenience or discomfort of any sort." Herbert M. Hart, Colonel, United States Marine Corps, who wrote an introduction to the reprint of Circular 9 commented that this statement on the ease of transport might not be entirely correct for the wounded of 1876 or those in Vietnam who took the litter route until faster evacuation means were at hand.

STERNBERG'S USE OF PACK ANIMALS FOR TRANSPORT OF WOUNDED

George Miller Sternberg, later to be Surgeon General of the United States in 1893, was involved in the Battle of the Clearwater, Idaho, July 11 and 12, 1877, against the Nez Perces Indians. Because he was recuperating from an extremely severe case of yellow fever, Sternberg was told that his special responsibility would be the care of the wounded and to remove wounded from the battlefield. Indians had a reputation of mistreating those who became their prisoners, so it was necessary to move the wounded to a safe place.

Dr. Sternberg moved the wounded and dead during the dark of night, attempting to find those who could be helped. The Indians were guarding the only water supply and snipers watched for any movements. After surveying the battlefield, Sternberg returned to the officers' tent and secured several volunteers to run the blockade of the water supply. All of them returned safely but had risked their lives in order to help their wounded comrades. Major Sternberg decided to operate on one man without moving him, using a candle behind a blanket held by two men. The Indians saw the light and let loose a burst of rifle fire. Dr. Sternberg finished the operation in the dark. The wounded man recovered.

When it came time to pursue the retreating Indians, Sternberg was left behind to transport the wounded to a hospital twenty-five miles away. The best mules and horses remained with the main forces. Also, only the wagons which were unsuitable for pursuit were left for Dr. Sternberg's use.

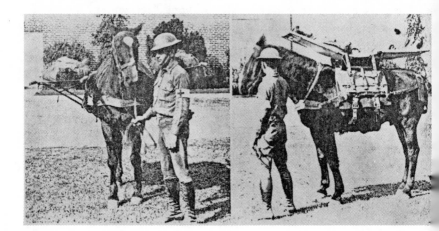

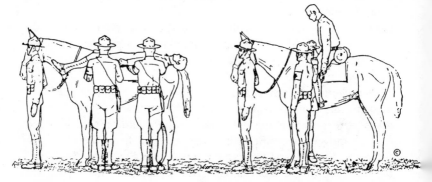

The illustrations above show American soldiers, circa the First World War, using pack animals for transporting the wounded.
TOP: The photo on the left shows the Carlisle cacolet; the photo on the right shows the 1st Division cacolet.
BOTTOM: This drawing demonstrates the method of placing a wounded soldier on a horse and carrying him astride.

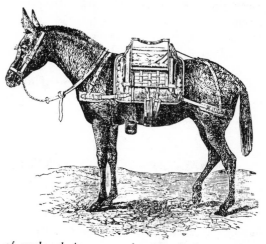

Side view of mule chair or cacolet attached to its pack-saddle.

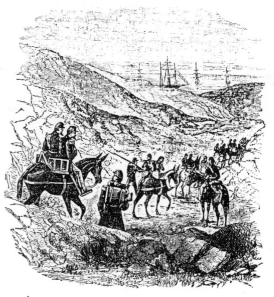

Illustration of a convoy of wounded being removed on mule-cacolets.

Having seen the Cheyennes use a type of carrier for their wounded, he built travois out of long lodge poles lashing one end of each pole to each side of a pack saddle. The other end dragged on the ground. Between the poles was suspended a wooden bridge with blankets on it or the blanket was used as a hammock. In this way, the wounded soldiers were transported to Grangeville where women helped to prepare food and located a building which could be used as a hospital.

DUNDONALD'S CAMEL AMBULANCE

Perhaps the most interesting contribution of Lord Dundonald to the comfort of his fellow soldiers is his camel ambulance. Besides being remarkably light and compact, this vehicle minimizes the terrible jog trot of the camel's gait, which to a wounded soldier is like the earthquakes of Vesuvius, the laboring of a tugboat in the British channel, the rack of a bucking mustang, and the jolts of a corduroy pike. The ambulance is shown in the illustrations both packed and in use.

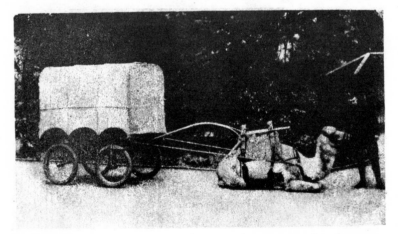

Lord Dundonald's camel ambulance as it appears when in use— it will accommodate two sick or wounded soldiers comfortably.

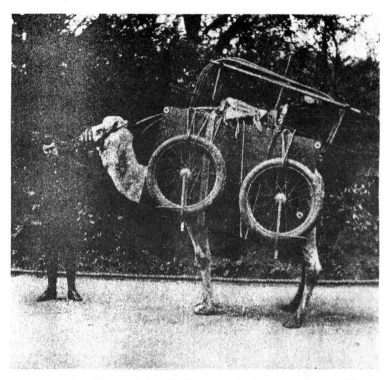

Lord Dundonald's camel ambulance packed for transport. (From photographs by Faulkner, London)

MOJAVE INDIAN LITTER
FOR CARRYING WOUNDED—1888

Charles Sewall, acting assistant Surgeon, U.S.A., in 1890, wrote about his new extemporaneous litter. While serving at Fort Mojave, Arizona Territory, in 1888, Dr. Sewall observed a wounded Mojave Indian who had been brought some seventeen miles in remarkably good condition by means of an unusual method of transportation. A wagon sheet of canvas was loosely tied at the ends to a long cottonwood pole. The ends of the pole were carried on the shoulders of two men. When these men

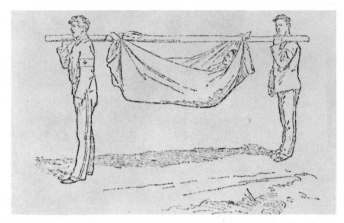

The illustration above was taken from an article by C. A. Sewall entitled "A New Extemporaneous Litter, Copied after the Mojave Method of Carrying the Wounded," which appeared in Medical Record, *1890.*

stood erect the wounded Indian was lying about two to four feet from the ground. The slightly flexed position of the body of the patient insured an easy ride.

Major Washington Matthews, Surgeon, U.S.A., suggested that a stone added to each corner of an army blanket by a stout cord would keep the blanket from slipping when tied to the pole. A nail or groove in the pole would also serve to keep the canvas from slipping toward the center.

6

Hospital Ambulances
After the Civil War—
1865 to 1900

Strangely enough the innovations in ambulance design took place during wartimes. After the wars the modes of carrying sick and wounded remained much the same with adaptations for civilian life. Many of the hospitals which were involved in caring for wounded soldiers during the Civil War continued the ambulance service for peacetime.

Following are some pictures of hospital ambulances which have been kept in the files of Hospital Histories and brought out to show on anniversaries and special occasions. The hospital ambulance in those times was a proud possession.

COMMERCIAL HOSPITAL, CINCINNATI—1865

Although Bellevue Hospital in New York claimed to have the first ambulance service which served the whole city in 1869, the records show that hospital ambulance service was introduced by the Commercial Hospital (now the Cincinnati General) in Cincinnati, Ohio, before 1865. The list of employees for the year ending February 28, 1866, names James R. Jackson, employee No. 27 as driver of ambulance at an annual salary of $360.

NEW YORK'S FIRST HOSPITAL
AMBULANCE SERVICE—1869

Dr. Edward B. Dalton was appointed Sanitary Superintendent of the newly organized New York Metropolitan Board of Health in 1866. Dr. Dalton had had extensive experience as an army

61

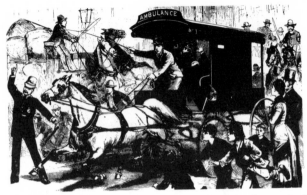

An engraving from 1881 shows the popular view of the ambulance racing through a city street. (Courtesy of National Library of Medicine, Bethesda, Maryland)

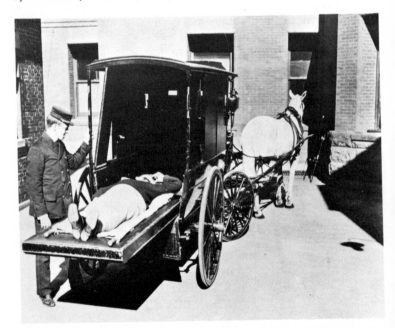

This is a picture of the ambulance of Presbyterian Hospital, New York City. It is similar in design to the Cincinnati ambulances. (Courtesy of National Library of Medicine, Bethesda, Maryland)

surgeon during the Civil War. When Bellevue was establishing a reception hospital in the lower city, he organized an ambulance service along military lines to provide for transport of patients. Bellevue claimed to have initiated the world's first ambulance service associated with a hospital, in 1869. However, it was later discovered that Cincinnati, Ohio had such a service in 1865. In July, 1869, a riot occurred in Elm Park, four miles from the hospital. According to the 1893 published account of Bellevue Hospital, the ambulance system was found to work with perfect smoothness in travelling to the scene of the riot and bringing wounded to the hospital. In 1870 there were 1401 ambulance calls, and in 1891 Bellevue responded to 4392 calls for an ambulance.

Dr. Dalton outlined a plan of service which was immediately adopted. A warden was appointed to see that the ambulances were in good order and fit for service. Each vehicle was to have a box beneath the driver's seat containing a quart of brandy, two tourniquets, six bandages, six small sponges, splint material, blankets, and a two ounce vial of persulphate of iron. Abbott-Downing company manufactured the ambulance.

Two surgeons were assigned to the ambulance corps after an examination as to their ability to handle emergencies. They were not attached to the regular house staff. Drivers of the ambulances received an annual salary of five hundred dollars, board and room. The vehicle was light weight, six hundred to eight hundred pounds. A moveable floor could be drawn out to receive the patient. The ambulance carried a stretcher, handcuffs, and strait jacket for the insane.

Stables for the horses were just north of the hospital, connected by telephone to the main building. A "drop" or "snap" harness was used enabling the ambulance to be ready in thirty seconds. It could then travel at the rate of one mile in five to eight minutes.

THE HAMMOCK VAN—1876

Richard Davy, Surgeon to the Westminster Hospital in 1876, wrote *Remarks on the Transit of Invalids.* He began his discourse

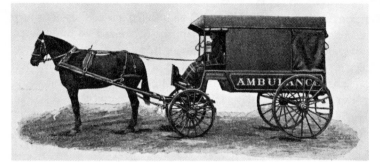

Bellevue Hospital Ambulance Number 3. From "An Account of Bellevue Hospital" edited by Robert J. Carlisle, M.D. and published in 1893 by the Society of the Alumni of Bellevue Hospital, New York.

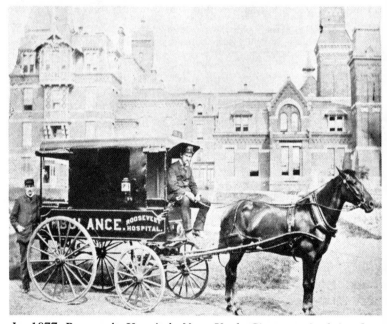

In 1877 Roosevelt Hospital, New York City, acquired its first ambulance. (Courtesy of National Library of Medicine, Bethesda, Maryland)

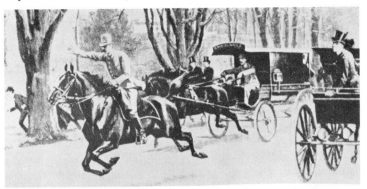

Mounted policeman clearing the way for an ambulance in New York City, 1881. From a Historical Sketch of New York University College of Medicine, by C. E. Heaton, M.D., 1941. (Courtesy of National Library of Medicine, Bethesda, Maryland)

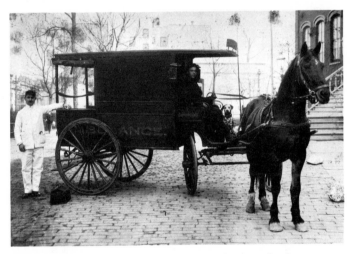

Dr. Isadore Faust, intern on ambulance duty at the front entrance of the original Lebanon Hospital. This building, located at Westchester and Cauldwell avenues in the East Bronx, New York, had been an Ursuline Convent. It was purchased in 1894 to start Lebanon Hospital. This photo was taken in 1911. (Courtesy of Mrs. Edith Faust)

by the comment, "The British public have practically evinced a far higher regard for the removal of valuable furniture than for the convenience of delicate Christians." Because of this situation, Dr. Davy introduced a "hammock van" for the convenience of invalids. The carriage could be drawn by one or two horses and permitted two hammocks to be swung, one above the other. It was furnished with strong springs, India rubber tires, seats for attendants, and a lavatory and its accompaniments. By employing this type of van, Dr. Davy claimed the patient was subjected to the least amount of inconvenience, although he might become slightly seasick. The van could be placed on a railway truck at the station and on reaching the end of the journey, could be taken off the truck and again attached to horses for the trip to its destination.

The van was made only by Messrs. Seydel and Company of Birmingham, England. In 1882, six years after his first article was published, Dr. Davy again directed his attention to the absolute necessity of improvement in carriages for the comfort of the patient and for the convenience of the surgeon in charge. This time he advocated the use of a three wheeled van, length nine feet, breadth four and a half feet, and height four and a half feet. This van was large enough to receive the patient's own bed if this seemed practical. He offered to exhibit the van to anyone interested.

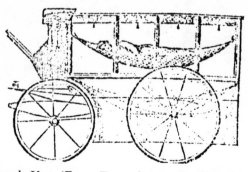

The Hammock Van (From Remarks on the Transit of Invalids *by Richard Davy, 1876)*

A HOSPITAL AMBULANCE—1878

W. H. Rideing (1853-1918) was an American journalist and author who wrote for the very popular *Harper's New Monthly Magazine.* In 1878, he wrote a description of "Hospital Life in New York." His comments were quite dramatic and probably reflected the middle-class view of the medical profession at that time.

Rideing told of his own experience one day when he was in the apothecary shop of the New York Hospital. He was conversing with a friend, Dr. Slaughter (an unfortunate name for a physician, Rideing comments), when an instrument on the wall began to ring insistently. The doctor explained that the ringing meant that an ambulance was wanted on Eighteenth Street. The apothecary shop opened into a courtyard at the side of a stable. A horse from the stable was rapidly harnessed to the ambulance. The surgeon in his special cap and uniform jumped in the back, the driver sprang on to the box alongside of Mr. Rideing, and the ambulance moved out into the street.

While the ambulance was speeding on its way, the driver and surgeon continually shouted at people to get out of the way. When pedestrians saw the word ambulance on the wagon, they immediately made room for this important carrier of relief to the suffering.

According to Rideing, the case was not very serious. A laborer had fallen and fractured his leg. However, the surgeon treated him with great concern. A stretcher (which the journalist thought was ingenious) was brought from the ambulance and the injured man was placed on it by two burly policemen. The stretcher consisted of a strip of canvas about three feet wide and seven feet long, with a tube at each side, through which the wooden carrying poles were slipped. The poles were braced at each end by iron cross bars which were easily detached.

The ambulance was backed up to the curb and a frame on casters was rolled from the back of the wagon to the curb. The stretcher was placed on it and pushed into the ambulance.

The ride to the hospital was more exciting than the one which they had on the way to the injured party. Now, everyone wanted to see the patient and the ambulance driver had an excuse to race for time, assuming all ambulance calls were lifesaving ones.

When the patient arrived at the hospital, the stretcher was placed on the bed and the poles were removed.

The city was divided into three police telegraph districts for the purpose of giving ambulance service. The hospitals with ambulances in 1878 were the New York, Roosevelt, and Bellevue Hospitals. When an accident was reported at a police station, it was immediately announced by telegraph to the hospital in the district.

AMBULANCE AT JEWISH HOSPITAL,
PHILADELPHIA, PENNSYLVANIA—1884

The horse-drawn ambulance service began at Jewish Hospital in 1884. This necessitated the improvement of stable facilities. In the first year, there were only twelve calls for its use. In 1894, ten years later, there were one hundred and fifty-six emergency cases. Many times it was used to convey sick or injured dignitaries to their homes or to the hospital.

In 1913, the hospital was fortunate to be able to buy an automobile ambulance.

THE LIVERPOOL AMBULANCE—1885

Captain William Joynson, Chairman of the Northern Hospital, Liverpool, England, reported to a Hospitals Association meeting held on April 15, 1885, the following information. At the close of 1882, he had made a voyage to America via the Cunard ship *Gallia*. Upon arriving in New York, an invalid aboard ship was removed from the ship by means of an ambulance carriage and taken .with every comfort to the hospital. This service was rendered upon the receipt of a telephone call to the hospital from the captain of the ship. Captain Joynson was so impressed with this

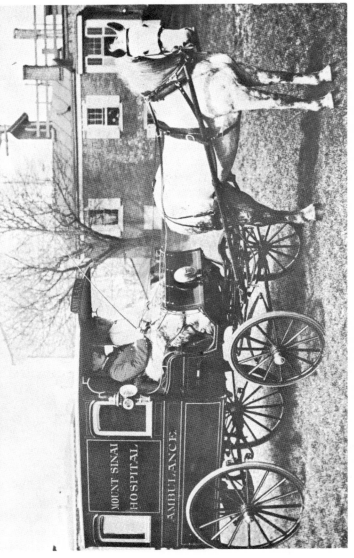

A forerunner of Mount Sinai Hospital's horse-drawn ambulance, shown in this photo taken around 1910, was the horse-drawn ambulance service begun at Jewish Hospital in Philadelphia in 1884. (Courtesy Albert Einstein Medical Center)

experience in New York that he had then established the perfect ambulance service in connection with the Liverpool Northern Hospital. He explained that the ambulances were really moving hospitals with a surgeon on the spot to render those services which might mean the difference between life and death.

Rapidity of action was ensured by the use of a patent American clip-harness. The harness was suspended from the ceiling, the saddle and collar were hung ready to be dropped into place. When the bell sounded the horse was placed under the shafts and the harness, saddle, and collar were immediately snapped on. The driver took the ambulance to the front of the hospital and picked up the surgeon, and, according to Captain Joynson, the moving hospital was on its way in two minutes.

The Liverpool ambulance was designed by Mr. John Furley of the St. John Ambulance Association and was built of English oak and American ash and birch. There were two stretchers in each carriage, both provided with telescopic handles. Medical appliances, splints, bandages, and other requisites were ready for use in each ambulance.

The ambulance in use was called about three times every two days. The time from call to departure was 2.14 minutes by day, and four minutes by night. Each journey from call to return, was eighteen minutes and thirty seconds.

This ambulance carried a selection of dressings, drugs, splints, and even a tracheotomy set so that there was intensive care from door to door.

ANNUAL COST

Driver's Wages (24 shillings per week)	66 pounds/ 6 shillings
Horse Hire (30 shillings per week)	78 pounds
Cottage for Driver (6 shillings per week)	11 pounds/14 shillings
Rent of Stable	20 pounds
Telephone	15 pounds/10 shillings
Livery for Driver	6 pounds/ 6 shillings
Insurance	4 pounds/10 shillings
Repairs	25 pounds
Total	227 pounds/ 6 shillings

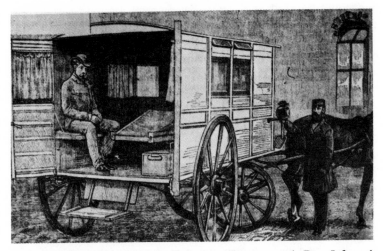

The Northern Hospital Ambulance. (Courtesy of Dr. John A. Ross, Consultant Radiologist, David Lewis Northern Hospital [formerly Northern Hospital,] Liverpool, England)

CHARITY HOSPITAL AMBULANCE—NEW ORLEANS

A. B. Miles wrote a letter to the *New Orleans Medical and Surgical Journal* which was printed on June 16, 1885. The letter described the ambulance service which Mr. Miles had organized.

The ambulance equipment of Eastern hospitals was thoroughly examined and the best features were incorporated into vehicles for the Charity Hospital. The carriages were built by Abbott-Downing Company of Concord, New Hampshire. They were very attractive with the words "Charity Hospital" in gold lettering on the sides. Each vehicle weighed sixteen hundred pounds and required a double team. It had a carriage finish and was mounted on easy springs. The body was made entirely of paneled wood lined with varnished maple. The interior was fitted with medicine chests, boxes for surgical apparatus, racks for splints, and hooks for lanterns. An easy bed trundled in and out

and could be used as a litter. There were separate springs for
the bed to rest on. The medicine chests contained "chloroform,
sulphuric ether, whiskey, brandy, carbolic acid, olive oil, ferri
ox. hydrat., Monsel's solution, dialysed iron, ergot, fl. ext. aqua
ammonia, solution ammon. carb., cosmoline, mustard, syrup
morph., sulph., tr. opii camph., hyperdermic tablets and syringe,
water, graduated glasses, one gallon of carron oil."

The surgical outfit consisted of the following: Complete
pocket case of instruments, extra Langenbeck's forceps, set of
three tourniquets, folding fracture box, two Liston's long splints,
wooden and tin splints for extremity fractures, bandages, charpie,
carbolized gauze, cotton padding, pillows, oakum, surgeon's lint,
sponges, tracheotomy tube, Nelaton's catheter, pus pans, water
bucket, etc.

The wagons having been constructed and equipped as above
described, and the fourteen Resident Students charged with the
special duty of "ambulance surgeons," the Charity Hospital ambulance service was organized by resolution of the Board of
Administrators, February 2, 1885.

Some of the specific ambulance runs reported are: March 2,
"Lady fell in open gutter and dislocated her shoulder and fractured her leg. Ambulance reached her and brought her to hospital in fifteen minutes; May 15, Mexican musician was shot on
the Exposition Grounds. Ambulance reached him in forty-five
minutes. He recovered and played concert for the benefit of the
Ambulance Fund, the proceeds of which was $693; March 3, a
Negro received a stabbing wound of the abdomen four and a
half inches in length, through which protruded the small bowel.
The ambulance surgeon arrived promptly, reduced the bowel,
sutured the wound and conveyed the patient to the hospital. He
recovered satisfactorily; June 7, the excursion train of the Mis-
sissippi Valley Railroad was derailed causing serious injuries
among the passengers. Ambulances were dispatched with seven
medical-staff members who superintended the conveyance of those
who chose to come to the hospital."

By a system of signals turned in from the fire boxes, located
in different parts of the city, the engineer of the fire department

could call an ambulance when it was needed. Mr. Miles claimed that the hospital ambulance service in New Orleans, within the five months of its existence, had become one of the most useful of the public charities.

THE AMBULANCE CHAIR

Mr. Hugh M. Smellie, M.B., C.M. (visiting surgeon to the Jarrow Memorial Hospital in 1891) recommended the ambulance chair seen here. Fig. 1 shows the chair with a subject in the act of being raised in a horizontal position; this position is particularly suitable for a person suffering from an injury to the thigh or hip. Fig. 2 shows the subject in what might be termed a sitting posture. Fig. 3, the patient is represented in a perpendicular position which is assumed for the purpose of raising or lowering a person through a narrow opening. When the disabled person has been raised or lowered to the required spot he need not be removed from the chair. The patient can be carried by simply removing the chair and slings from the block and then, by passing a hand spike or pole through the ring for the slings, two men can conveniently move the patient (Fig. 1). The chair can also be made use of in shipwrecks in cases where a sick or disabled person has to be brought ashore.

The inventors and proprietors were Messrs. John F. and Thomas H. Singleton, 143 Albert Road, Jarrow, England.

INVALID COACH—1901

The invalid coach as pictured in the *Buffalo Medical Journal* for September, 1901, offered residents of the city "transportation without the publicity of the common ambulance." After the patient was in the carriage and the back closed, there was nothing to show that it was an ambulance. The coach had room for a six-foot bed with air mattress and pillow and seating accommodations for two persons accompanying the patient. The patient reclining at the rear of the vehicle is ready for placement inside.

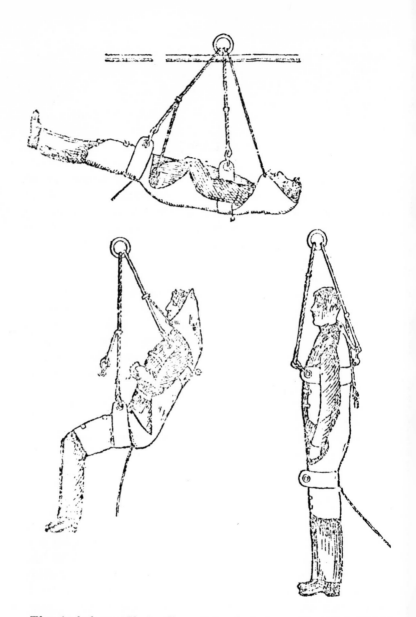

The Ambulance Chair. (From "An Ambulance Chair," in British Medical Journal, *1891)*

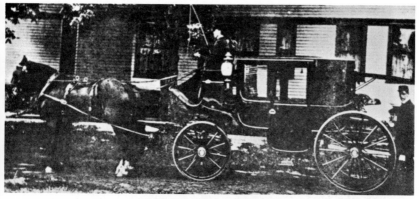

Invalid coach, 1901.

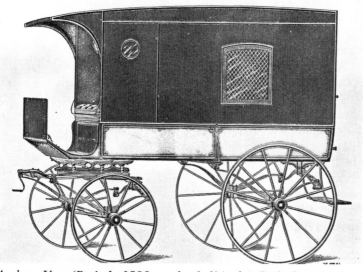

Asylum Van (Period: 1890; scale, half-inch) Built for use in a New Jersey town, this van was used in conveying inmates of an insane asylum. One barred window on each side; single door in back with a barred window on each side. Lengthwise seats inside. Body 48 inches wide; 22-inch door. (Courtesy of National Library of Medicine, Bethesda, Maryland)

RED CROSS AMBULANCE OF 1898

Ambulances marked with a red cross were furnished by the German Army Quartermaster Corps as early as 1870 in the Franco-Prussian War. However, the first effort of a civilian corps to provide ambulances at any battlefront was during the period of the Spanish-American War. Six ambulances were sent to Cuba in 1898. Although Clara Barton had become interested in the Cuban revolt in 1897, she avoided provoking international complications which might lead to war between the United States and Spain. After the declaration of war against Spain on April 25, 1898, the U. S. Government officially accepted the aid of the American Red Cross. A committee was formed under the title of "First New York Ambulance Equipment Society." Its purpose was to purchase and equip ambulances. The Society raised money and purchased the vehicles from the Studebaker Brothers Manufacturing Company of South Bend, Indiana.

Miss Barton travelled to Cuba to survey the needs there. Six ambulances were shipped to Havana by Stephen Barton, Clara's nephew, who was chairman of the "President's Committee for Cuban Relief." Later the Committee sent forty mules to Miss Barton along with fodder and harnesses. Owing to the delay in unloading, the six ambulances could be put to no use in Cuba, and they were returned to New York after the signing of the armistice on October 24, 1898. In November, 1898, official protest was made by the Red Cross to the U.S. government for its delayed delivery of the ambulances and for having seized ten thousand dollars worth of supplies.

On July 23, 1898, two ambulances and mules were shipped from Tampa, Florida, to Puerto Rico. These proved of great value in emergency cases requiring quick transportation of soldiers and supplies. When the station closed in Puerto Rico, the vehicles were sold to a Mr. Hersey for two hundred dollars.

The Red Cross Relief Station at Long Island City was opened on August 29. Two ambulances were supplied by Auxiliary No. 1. The station was used as a stopping point for soldiers too sick to

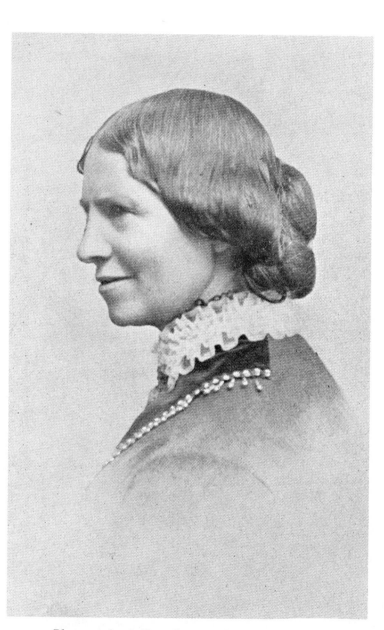

Photograph of Clara Barton taken about 1884.

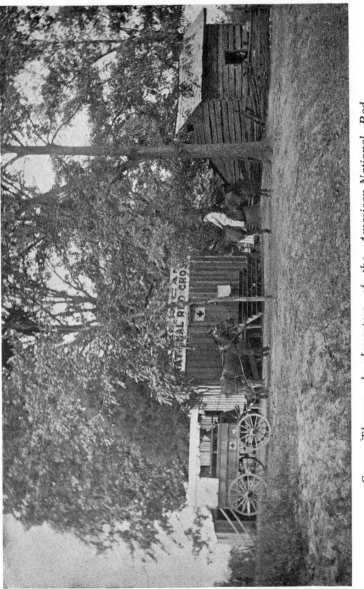

Camp Thomas, headquarters of the American-National Red Cross at Chickamauga Park, Georgia, 1898.

be transported long distances. With the removal of troops, the relief station was closed and the ambulances were transferred to two convalescent homes.

In June, 1898, Red Cross work was started at Camp Thomas, Chickamauga Park, Georgia. An ambulance and mules were sent to the Georgia station. When these facilities were closed, the ambulance was sent to Clara Barton for her use in Glen Echo. It was this particular ambulance which was restored for display in the Smithsonian's Museum of History and Technology.

The original manufacturer's plate bearing the name Studebaker Brothers Manufacturing Company, South Bend, Indiana, remains on the ambulance. It was intended to be drawn by a pair of oxen or mules. The vehicle is eight and a half feet high over all, seven feet wide including the wheels, and eleven feet long. The floor is thirty-eight inches from the ground, and the sides are twenty-seven inches. The canvas is supported by seven hoops which are connected with crossbars. The tailgate is thirteen and a half inches high, and the back step is thirty-six inches long and nine inches wide. The diameter of the back wheels is forty-nine inches and of the front wheels thirty-seven and a half inches. The hubs are seven inches in diameter. A foot lever at the driver's right operates the rear-wheel brakes. A water cask is under the driver's seat. The body rests on platform springs. This type of ambulance was equipped with four stretchers, two at the top and two at the bottom.

First Red Cross Relief Boat on American Waters—1884

Clara Barton describes the 1884 Ohio River floods in her book *The Red Cross, A History of this Remarkable International Movement in the Interest of Humanity,* published in 1898. One thousand miles of the Ohio River flooded its banks in February, 1884. The government appropriated several thousand dollars for relief. Clara Barton traveled to Pittsburgh, the head of the Ohio River, to observe the situation herself. Local Red Cross Societies were telegraphed that Cincinnati, Ohio, would be headquarters and that money and supplies should be sent there.

In Miss Barton's own words she tells about the flood in Cincinnati.

> The surging river had climbed up the bluffs like a devouring monster and possessed the town; large steamers could have plied along its business streets; ordinary avocations were abandoned. Bankers and merchants stood in its relief houses and fed the hungry populace, and men and women were out in boats passing baskets of food to pale, trembling hands stretched out to reach it from third-story windows of the stately blocks and warehouses of that beautiful city. Sometimes the water soaked away the foundations and the structure fell with a crash and was lost in the floods below; in one instance seven lives went out with the falling building; and this was one city, and probably the best protected and provided locality in a thousand miles of thickly populated country.

A flood of supplies began to come in to Cincinnati. All available help was needed for the care and distribution of the gifts. The government provided neither fuel nor clothing. It was midwinter and a cyclone swept away whole villages in a single night. The inhabitants escaped homeless and without clothes or food. Hail encased the country in sleet and ice. Coal mines were inundated so that fuel could not be obtained.

A new steamer of four-hundred tons was chartered and laden with clothing and coal. The Red Cross flag was hoisted. Amid surging waters and crashing ice and the wrecks of towns and villages the *Josh V. Throop* set out from Evansville, Indiana, the first Red Cross relief boat to float on American waters. Not only were supplies being taken to those who needed them, but the sick and wounded were transported to facilities where they could be cared for.

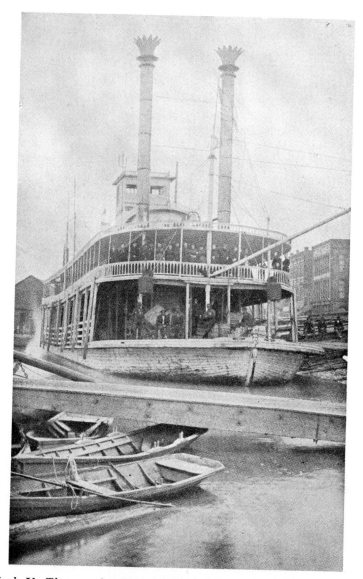

Josh V. Throop, the first steamer used in the United States by the American Red Cross, 1884.

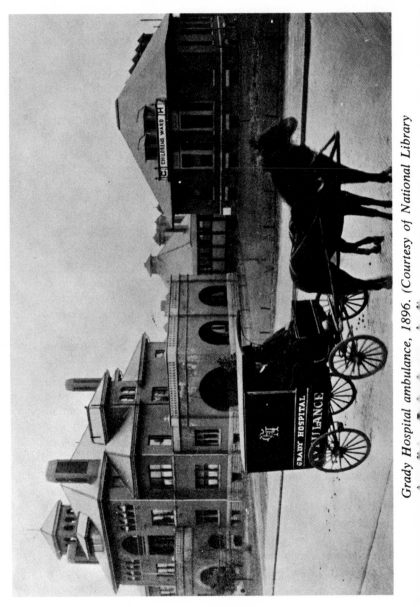

Grady Hospital ambulance, 1896. (Courtesy of National Library

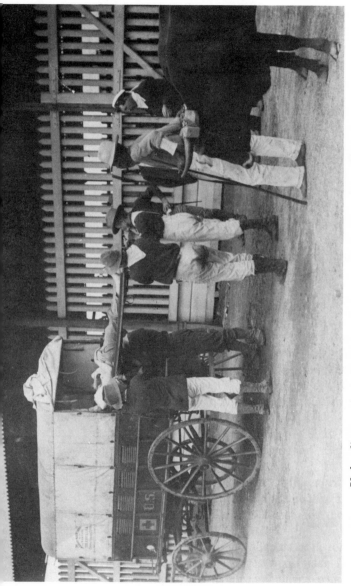

Unloading patients at the wharf for transfer from an ox-drawn ambulance train to the U.S. Hospital Ship Relief at Mayaguez, Puerto Rico. Photo, ca. 1898, from an album on the U.S. War of 1898. (Courtesy of National Library of Medicine, Bethesda, Maryland)

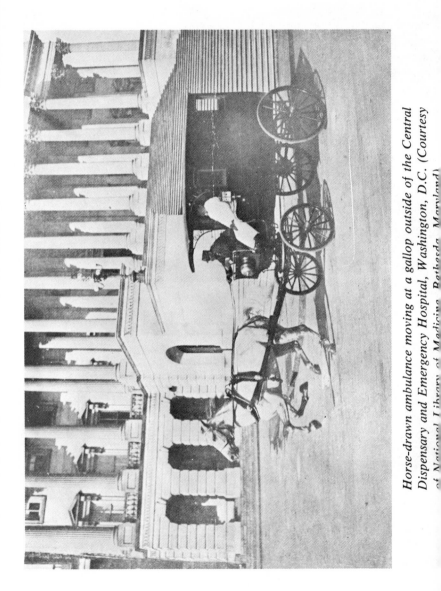

Horse-drawn ambulance moving at a gallop outside of the Central Dispensary and Emergency Hospital, Washington, D.C. (Courtesy of National Library of Medicine, Bethesda, Maryland).

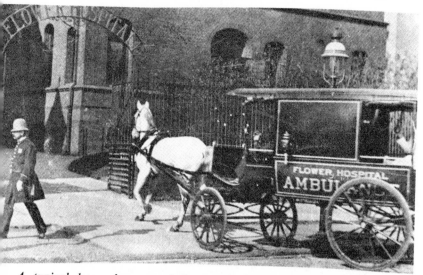

A typical horse-drawn ambulance at the turn of the century. This particular one belongs to Flower Hospital, New York City. There is a nurse riding in attendance.

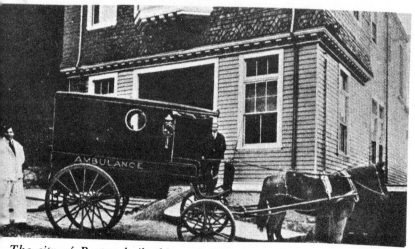

The city of Boston built this ambulance station in 1899 on the grounds of the Carney Hospital.

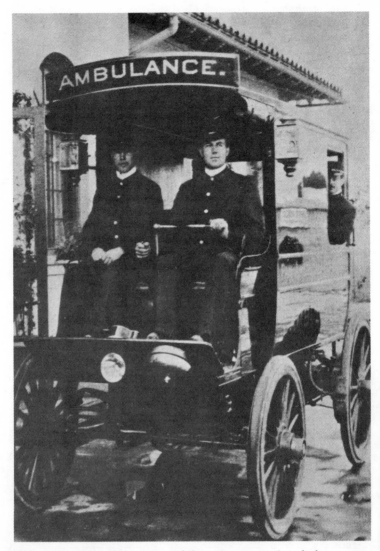

With the coming of the automobile a new type of ambulance came on the scene. This ambulance brought President McKinley to the hospital after he was shot at the Buffalo Exhibition in 1901. (Courtesy of National Library of Medicine, Bethesda, Maryland)

7

Motor Ambulances and
Other Ingenious Devices

The automobile was a product of an age when many individuals and industries were experimenting in the attempt to achieve locomotion with the different power devices that were being developed.

In the late 1800s several inventors were successful in creating automobiles and other self-propelled vehicles.

Following are some of these ingenious inventions as they were used to carry sick and wounded.

The *New York Herald,* February 24, 1899, printed the following news item: "The first automobile ambulance ever constructed was presented today to Michael Reese Hospital of this city [Chicago]. It was built in Chicago and was the gift of five prominent businessmen. The ambulance weighs sixteen hundred pounds and its speed approximates sixteen miles per hour."

A year later, the following notice appeared in the same newspaper: "A motor ambulance is the latest thing in horseless vehicles, and the one delivered last week to Saint Vincent's Hospital, New York City, by Frederick R. Wood and Son is said by the makers to be the first automobile ambulance to be built and put into service in this or any other country. 'An ambulance of this kind,' the manufacturer says, 'possesses many advantages over its horse-drawn prototype. A greater speed is attainable; and there is more ease and safety for the patient; it may be stopped within its own length when running at full speed, and on account of its weight, it runs with greater smoothness.' "

These first motor ambulances were electrically powered. They

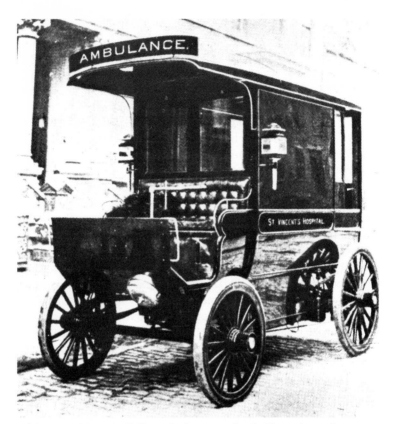

*The second automobile ambulance to be built and put into serv-
ice in this country. It was delivered to Saint Vincent's Hospital,
New York City, in 1900.*

were propelled by two horsepower motors suspended on the rear
axle. The vehicles could be driven at six, nine, or thirteen miles
per hour for twenty to thirty miles. A speaking tube extended
from driver to doctor for communication. Mountings were brass.
The litters slid out the rear for loading and unloading. Ten
candlepower electric lights were used inside and outside.

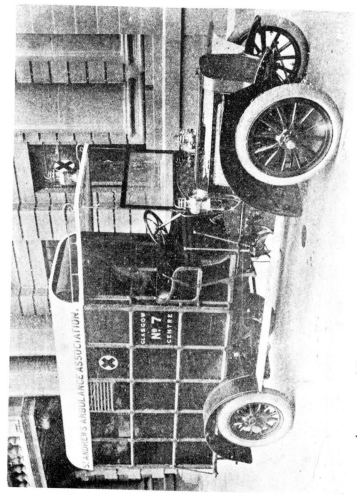

An automobile ambulance which was internally heated by the exhaust gases used in Glasgow, Scotland, for Saint Andrew's Ambulance Association.

PALLISER'S AMBULANCE AUTOMOBILE—1905

Major Palliser of the Canadian Militia introduced the idea of the Ivel-armored Red Cross Motor intended for service at the firing line. It was a three-wheeled vehicle with an eighteen horse-power, twin-cylinder, gasoline motor. The tractor was heavy, encased in bullet proof steel shields. Flaps opened outward protecting the ambulance staff when the vehicle was stationary. The protected area was nine feet wide by seven feet high.

The staff consisted of an engineer and a driver. The ambulance covered three to six miles an hour over rough ground. One of the

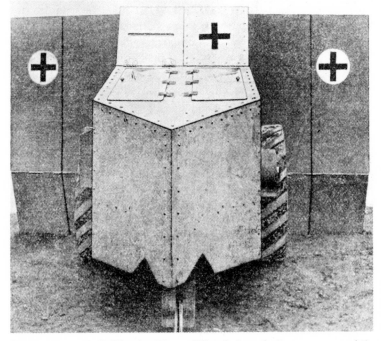

Front view of Palliser's Three Wheeled ambulance automobile. (Photograph from Scientific American, *volume 92, February 18, 1905)*

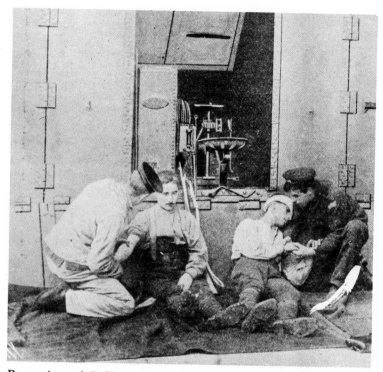

Rear view of Palliser's Three Wheeled ambulance automobile. *(Photograph from* Scientific American, *volume 92, February 18, 1905)*

disadvantages of this armored car was that gasoline fuel was not easily acquired on the battlefield.

When not in use the motor and driving mechanism could be disengaged and the car could be used as a stationary engine for generating electricity for illuminating the hospital tent.

STREETCAR AMBULANCE

This streetcar ambulance was used in Bahia, Brazil. There are five compartments. The one in the center is a fumigating com-

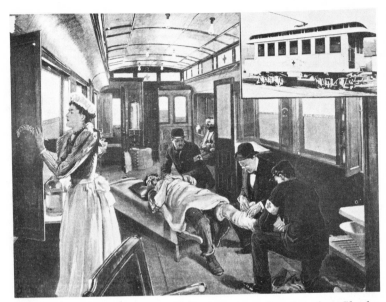

A trolley ambulance car. Halftone of a drawing by Charles Broughton and Photoinset from Harper's Weekly, *vol. 39:268 (March 23, 1895). (Courtesy of National Library of Medicine, Bethesda, Maryland)*

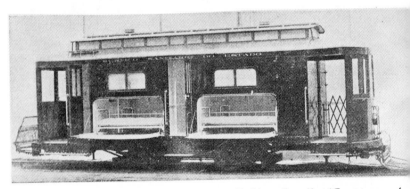

A streetcar ambulance used in Bahia, Brazil. (Courtesy of Scientific American)

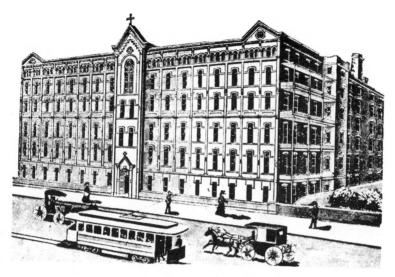

The streetcar ambulance (above and below) which was used in St. Louis, Missouri, in 1894. (Courtesy of Scientific American, *1913)*

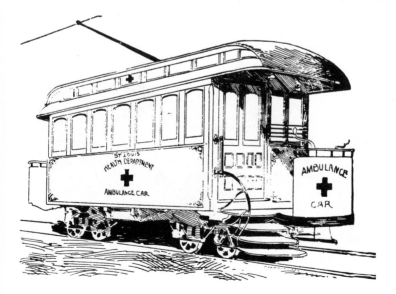

partment and nurse's room. Two iron beds are supplied with rubber-tired rollers, springs, and regular mattresses.

In 1894, St. Louis, Missouri had a street car ambulance which was able to travel to all sixteen infirmaries in the city.

GERMAN AMBULANCE TRAIN—1902

In 1902 a German ambulance train was in use for railway accidents. The train housed an operating room with a table, reclining chairs, and eight removable beds which were used as litters.

Railroad surgeons lived in the vicinity of the railway station where the ambulance train was sidetracked. Even the fast limited trains were ordered to give way to the surgeons and were sidetracked to let the ambulance train through.

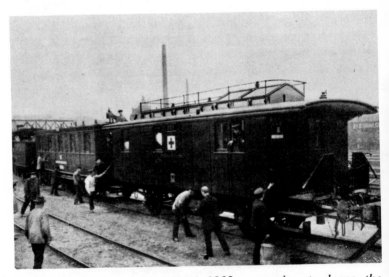

A German ambulance train of 1902, preparing to leave the station. (Courtesy of Scientific American, *1902)*

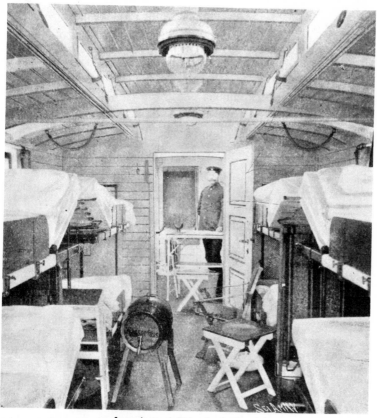

Interior of Hospital Car.

VELOCIPEDE AMBULANCE

An ambulance velocipede was patented in the United States and used at the Royal Charité Hospital, Berlin, in the late 1800s. Many of the disadvantages of the horse-drawn vehicle were thought to be overcome. The litter had a canvas covering, adjustable headrest and mattress. The bed rested on springs supported

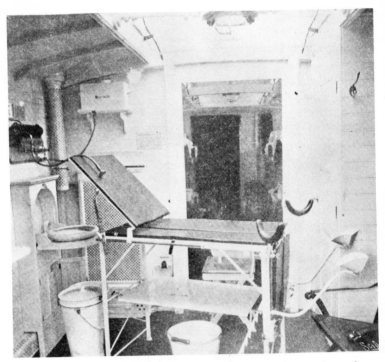

*An interior view of the hospital car and operating section, show-
ing the operating table.*

by bearings, the vehicle ran on five wheels with pneumatic tires.
The four rear wheels supported the body of the ambulance. The
front wheel was the guiding one, propelled by two persons. The
man in front was the driver; the man in the rear watched the
patient through the rear window. There were two side windows
which admitted light and air. The inside was lit by electric
lights. A box beneath the bed held medicine, bandages, and
instruments. The vehicle could be widened for two litters.

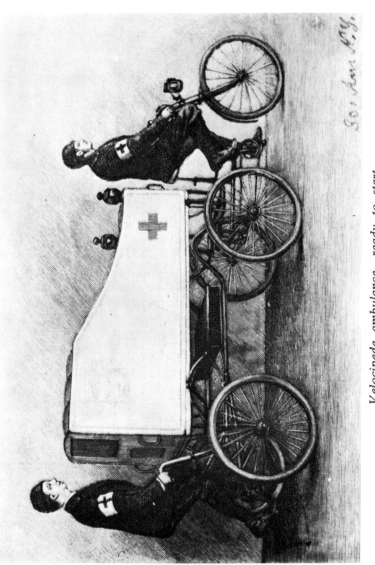

Velocipede ambulance—ready to start.

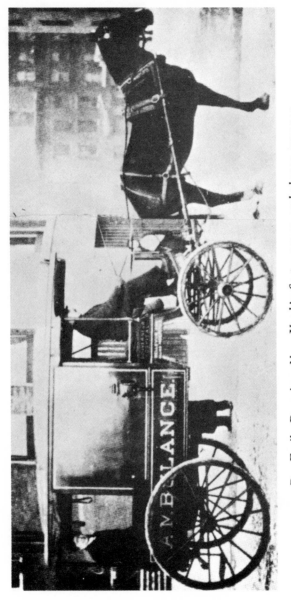

Dr. Emily Dunning, New York's first woman ambulance surgeon, in front of Gouverneur Hospital.

8

Drs. Dunning and Crawford—
First Women Ambulance Surgeons

Dr. Emily Dunning, intern at Gouverneur Hospital in New York City, took her first ambulance call on June 30, 1903. Her male superiors at the hospital had tormented her with tales of the dangers of riding the ambulance. Emily was determined to show that the female was not the weaker sex. She prepared herself mentally and physically to take her turn at riding on the back of a horse-drawn ambulance, pulled by wildly galloping horses. She even had a special uniform designed by V. Ballard and Sons of Boston. It was a two-piece outfit of navy blue serge lined with satin. It had a fitted waist and was military in style. The skirt came to the ankles but was made so that stepping up and down from the ambulance was not impeded. Pockets were cleverly hidden all through the uniform. A Mackintosh jacket was designed for wear in the cold weather.

The ambulance drivers were very helpful to Dr. Dunning. Their experience gave them the ability to judge which victims were real emergencies. Emily learned to hang on to the leather straps at the back of the ambulance as the vehicle flew along the streets.

After Dr. Dunning completed her residency at Gouverneur a delegation of ambulance drivers, policemen, and citizens of the Lower East Side presented her with a token of their appreciation in the form of a plaque.

Dr. Mary M. Crawford was Brooklyn's first ambulance surgeon. In 1908, she served as surgeon on a horse-drawn ambulance while interning at Williamsburg Hospital in Brooklyn, New York.

At the outbreak of World War I, Dr. Crawford went to France to serve at the American Ambulance Hospital at Neiully-sur-Seine.

TESTIMONIAL
from the
Citizens of New York,
the Police of the 7th, 12th, and 13th precincts,
and the Ambulance Drivers of Gouverneur Hospital
to
DR. EMILY DUNNING
upon her retirement, January 1, 1905, as
Chief of Staff of Gouverneur Hospital, New York

Dr. Dunning
for two years served the hospital and the people of New York in a manner that has won the admiration and esteem of her fellow-workers and all those with whom she has been brought in contact. Her wonderful skill, conscientious and untiring efforts, charm of manner, devotion to her patients, extreme kindness and consideration for all who labored with her, have endeared her to all.

AS THE ONLY WOMAN AMBULANCE SURGEON IN THE WORLD
she has won distinction that is world-wide and brought honor, not only upon herself but upon her sex, her profession, Gouverneur Hospital and the City of New York.

We hope and pray that the future may hold happiness and additional honors in store for her, and *Our best wishes* follow her in her new labors.

9

World War I
Ambulance Services

At the beginning of World War I, horse ambulances were used for battlefield transportation of wounded. However, adaptations of the automobile ambulance soon began to be used also. And during this war, the airplane was used. The airplanes were very small at that time, so they could accommodate only one or two patients.

According to the *United States Military Manual* (fourth edition, Medico-Military History) when war was declared on Germany by the United States, the medical department began a tremendous expansion. The Medical Reserve Corps and the American Red Cross had been in existence and were of great aid.

The French Army made a request of the medical department of the United States army for an ambulance service. A commissioned Ambulance Service Corps was established and sent to France.

Following are some of the illustrations for carrying wounded found in the *Military Medical Manual*. The ambulance company is described, and some of the motor transports used for ambulance service are pictured.

The Straker-Squire motor ambulance van was the first motor ambulance used by the British army, 1906. It was used for the first time in summer maneuvers (1907) when it was attached to a military hospital in Oxford. For the duration of the exercises it operated between there and the big military camps set up at Thame and Aylesbury. While in use, it attracted much attention.

The Boulant mobile surgery was of French design and used from 1912-18. What made this vehicle different from other motor-

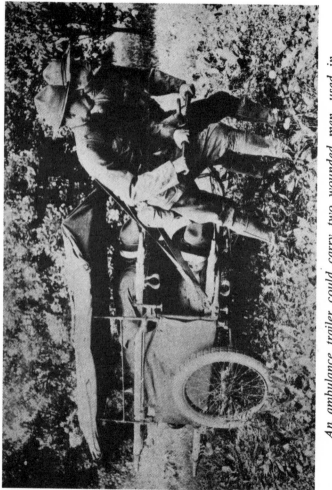

An ambulance trailer could carry two wounded men, used in World War I.

ized ambulances of its time was that it was a fully equipped mobile surgery unit. Used by the French Army Medical Service *(Service de Santé)*, it was built by Schnieder on the same Boulant chassis as used for Paris buses. It had a forty horsepower engine, solid rubber tires, twin rear wheels, and could travel at a speed of thirty kilometers per hour.

To make an easy entry for stretcher bearers, full-width double doors were fitted at the back of the body with wide steps. The body was divided into three compartments. In the rear, the entrance lobby contained a two-hundred liter water tank, wash basins and linen, and medical cabinets. The middle section formed an operating theater about twelve feet long and seven and a half feet wide, complete with operating table and electric light. The front compartment held the sterilizers. When the vehicle was stationary, folded tenting—which was afixed to each side of the body—was erected to form reception areas for patients with minor injuries or those awaiting attention.

The mobile surgery unit was prohibitively expensive and few were constructed. However, during WWI similar vehicles were constructed which were adapted from Paris buses. They were used primarily on the Western Front.

The Commer First Aid Van, which carried medical stores and stretchers to supply first aid posts, operated from casualty clearing stations as a mobile first aid post. Some were altered to be used as horse ambulances while others were only rigged with horsebox bodies.

The vehicle had a twenty-five horsepower four-cylinder engine and a Lindley gearbox.

The body was similar to a van but had slatted upper sides. There was a full-depth door which swung down creating a ramp for the injured animals, of which it could carry two. The horse ambulance version of the Commer carried extra veterinary supplies as well as slings and tackle for moving injured animals. The first aid van was usually accompanied by a medical officer or medical attendants.

French automobiles made military history on September 9, 1914. All the taxis in Paris were commandeered by the French army to rush the French 62nd Division to Marne to halt the enemy's threat to surround Paris. The Renault Paris taxis were soon adapted for other work as well; the saloon bodywork was removed and a simple framework body replaced it, arranged to hold stretchers.

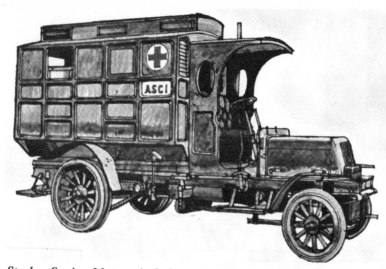

Straker-Squire Motor Ambulance Van, 1906-08, Great Britain.

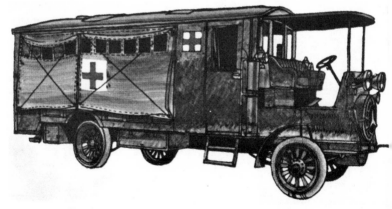

Boulant Mobile Surgery, 1912-18, France.

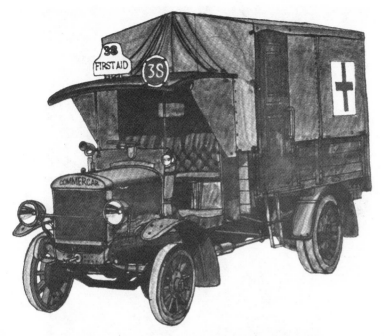

Commer Ambulance, 1916-18, Great Britain.

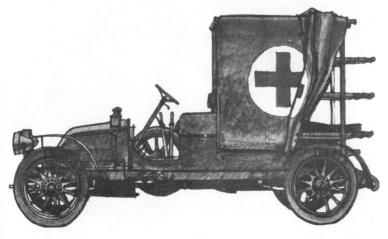

Renault Ambulance, 1914-18, France. (Courtesy C. Ellis, Military Transport of World War I, *Macmillan Company, 1970)*

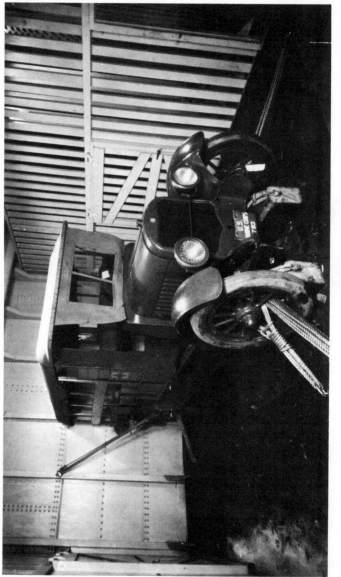

U.S. Navy-Marine Corps field ambulance "stowed for sea" aboard hospital ship Relief Feb. 1921. (Courtesy of James W. Wengert)

THE AIRPLANE AMBULANCE

During the First World War aviation rapidly passed from the experimental stage to that of a powerful arm of the military service without having had the opportunity of being applied to commercial uses. The war surplus of airplanes after the war easily met the demand and no new designing took place for several years.

The actual designing of airplanes as ambulances did not take place until the late 1920s or early 30s.

In 1929 the Air Corps had three Cox-Klemin planes which were designed for ambulance service. These planes had a speed of one-hundred miles an hour, carried six hours of fuel, and transported two litter patients, pilot, and attendant.

This is the first Air Ambulance used at Barksdale Field, Louisiana in 1933-34. It was an experimental model. Barksdale Field was the advanced training base of the Air Corps, U.S. Army.

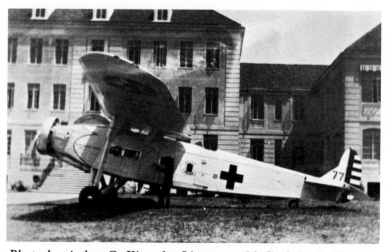

Photo by Arthur G. King, 1st Lieutenant Medical Corps Reserve Army of the United States, stationed at Barksdale Field as Assistant Surgeon.

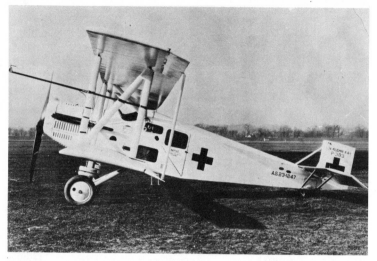

A photo of an airplane ambulance used in 1918. (Courtesy of National Library of Medicine, Bethesda, Maryland)

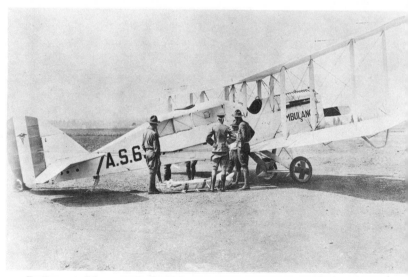

Patient and four stretcher bearers at an airplane ambulance, 1918. (Courtesy of National Library of Medicine, Bethesda, Maryland)

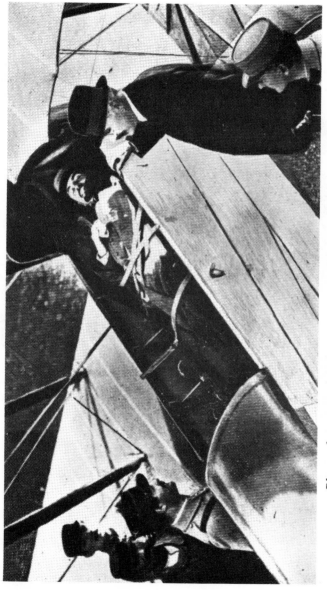

Photo demonstrating how a wounded person would be transported by airplane. A practice run at Villacoublay, France. (Courtesy Daily Mail, London, England)

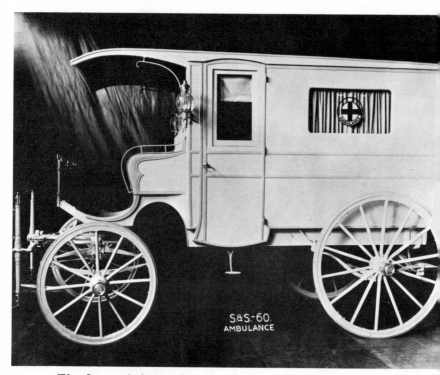

S&S-60.
AMBULANCE

The first ambulances built by the Hess and Eisenhardt Company appeared in 1890. They had one lantern, a stretcher, and two seats for attendants. The ambulance pictured was built in 1891. The trademark of "S & S" refers to the original owners of the company, Sayers and Scovill. (Courtesy of the Hess & Eisenhardt Co., Rossmoyne [Cincinnati], Ohio)

10

An Ambulance Builder,
an Ambulance Service,
and an Ambulance Association

HESS AND EISENHARDT—AMBULANCE BUILDERS

The Hess and Eisenhardt Company, Cincinnati, Ohio, is known the world over for its ambulances, hearses, and custom built cars. It is the world's oldest builder of ambulances and funeral cars. In 1937, the company sold the first air-conditioned ambulance built in America. Ambulances are now built in three sizes, for one, two, and four patients.

The firm began building carriages in 1876 as the Sayers and Scovill Company using the trademark "S & S." The trademark is still being used. In 1891, two office boys were hired, Emil Hess and Charles A. Eisenhardt, Sr. Later the sons of these men were Willard Hess, president of the company and Charles A Eisenhardt, Jr., chairman of the board.

Custom cars are less and less in demand but the market for ambulances is growing rapidly. Using Cadillac chassis, ambulances and hearses take about three months to build. They are noted for their individualized trim and high quality of finish. The company built its first ambulance in 1890. It had one lantern, a stretcher, and two crude seats for attendants. The seats were padded and could be let down from the wall.

Today's ambulance is a closed car with a commercial-sized oxygen tank that has a seven to eight hour supply. There is plenty of space for the attendant to move about. There is air-conditioning; medicine cabinets, roof lights and a two-way radio are also standard equipment. H & E officials believe that an ambulance should be a pre-hospital emergency room. Mr. Eisenhardt comments that fire-fighting equipment is up to date. How much more important is it that life-saving ambulances be fitted with the latest and best equipment!

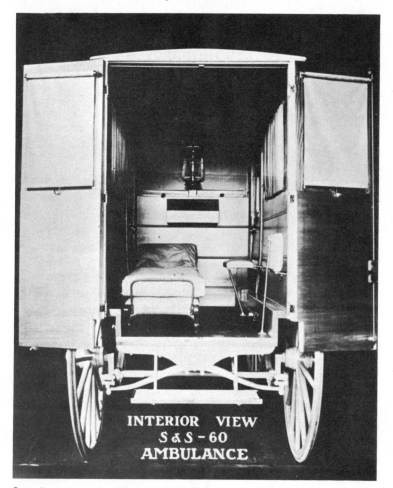

Interior view of a Hess and Eisenhardt ambulance built in 1895. (Courtesy of Hess & Eisenhardt Co.)

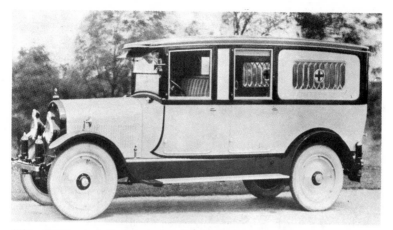

This 1923 model ambulance boasted having airsprings over the bumper for smoother riding. The interior had also been expanded for greater movement within. (Courtesy of Hess & Eisenhardt Co.)

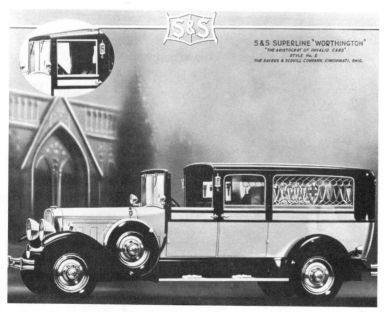

(Courtesy of Hess & Eisenhardt Co.)

BUCK AMBULANCE SERVICE, PORTLAND, OREGON, CELEBRATES SIXTY YEARS OF SERVICE

Ben C. Buck, Sr. and Frank Shephard started an ambulance service in 1913 in Portland, Oregon. They purchased one Speedwell and one Cadillac coach and formed the Portland Ambulance Service.

In 1915, Seattle called for help to start an ambulance service. A toss of a coin decided that Frank Shepherd would go to Seattle. Ben Buck was then sole owner of the Portland Company.

Mr. Buck donated one of the few motorized ambulances to the federal government at the outbreak of the First World War.

In 1942, Buck Ambulance became the first ambulance service in the country to carry oxygen as standard equipment. The Kaiser Shipyards in Portland found that many workers were being overcome by toxic gases. The need for oxygen before the victim reached the hospital led to the installation of oxygen in the Buck ambulances.

After the war, Buck initiated two-way radio operations between the main office and the ambulance. In the early 1950s the Buck Ambulance Service purchased a twin engine Cessna Box Car and thus became the first flying ambulance service in the Pacific Northwest.

In 1962, Barney Buck, Jr. and Lee Cox formed Century 21 Ambulance to serve the Seattle World's Fair.

An Emergency Medical Technician's training program for ambulance attendants was started by Buck in 1965. The first Cardiac Technicians' training and coronary care mobile unit was started by Buck in 1969. B. C. Buck, Sr. was the third person in acute cardiac distress to be saved by the cardiac team.

SAINT JOHN AMBULANCE ASSOCIATION

In 1877, the Order of Saint John decided to form the Saint John Ambulance Association to train personnel in first aid to minister to the sick and wounded in war, as well as in peacetime.

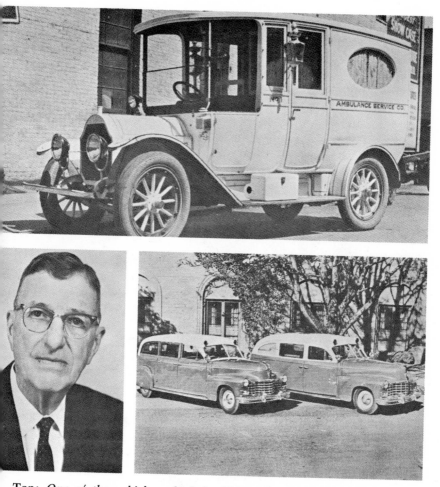

Top: *One of the vehicles which in 1913 gave Portland its first motorized ambulance service.* Left: *Ben C. Buck, Sr., who began his ambulance service in 1913.* Right: *With the opening of the World's Fair in 1962, Barney Buck, Jr., and Lee Cox formed "Century 21 Ambulance" using vehicles like the Cadillac pictured.*

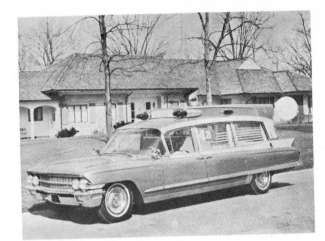

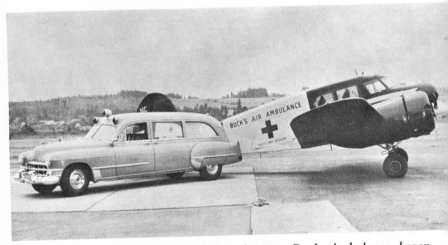

Top: *"Immediately following the war Buck Ambulance began another innovation in the ambulance industry: two-way radios."* Bottom: *"With a twin engine Cessna, Buck Ambulance initiated the first flying ambulance service in the Pacific Northwest."*

The principle objective of this Association was first, "the instruction of pupils in treatment of injured persons" and second, "spread of useful ambulance material."

The Association was ridiculed at first but this attitude changed when the Grand Prior Of the Order, Edward, Prince of Wales (later King Edward VII), asked for a guard of honor of men in Saint John uniform. Facing members of the press, he said, "Gentlemen, this is a good uniform. I believe much good will come of it."

In 1883, the Invalid Transport Corps was established. In 1898, a permanent Ambulance Station was established in the church-yard of Saint Clement Danes, later removed to Uxbridge.

In 1887, the Saint John Ambulance Brigade was created. This brigade has given innumerable services to the public. They have also published books and set up training classes.

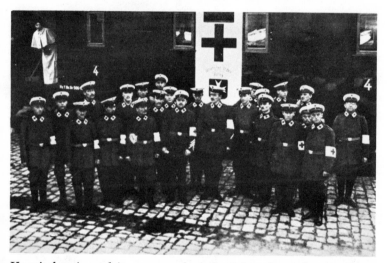

Hospital train and its personnel of the Johanniterorden, *or Prussian Order of Saint John during the World War. (From Edgar Erskine Hume,* Medical Work of the Knights Hospitallers of Saint John of Jerusalem, *Baltimore: Johns Hopkins University Press, 1940)*

11

Military Ambulances During World War II

The care of the sick and wounded on the field of battle reached its zenith during World War II. The following chart shows the organization of an ambulance company.

THE AMBULANCE COMPANY

There are three motorized companies in the ambulance battalion. They are designated as Company D, Company E, and Company F, respectively.

Organization. The ambulance company is organized into a company headquarters and two platoons.

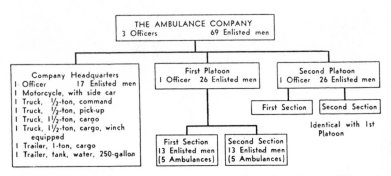

Suggested functional Organization of the Ambulance (Motor) Company, Medical Regiment.

118

Functions. The principal functions of the ambulance company are:

The transportation of casualties from collecting stations.

When practicable, the transportation of casualties from regimental aid stations, battalion aid stations, or other advanced loading posts to the clearing station.

The movement of non-transportable cases to the surgical hospital when the latter is located in the vicinity of the clearing station.

The transmission of messages along ambulance routes.

The transportation of medical personnel and supplies forward to medical installations being evacuated.

Command. The ambulance company is an integral part of the ambulance battalion. Its employment rests with the battalion commander, subject to the orders of the regimental commander.

When an ambulance company or a detachment thereof is attached to an advance, flank, or rear guard or to a detached force, the command thereof while so attached passes to the commander of the security detachment or detached force.

Company headquarters. Company headquarters consists of such commissioned and enlisted personnel as is required for the command, administration, and supply of the company as a whole.

Platoons. Both platoons of the ambulance company are identical in organization, equipment, and transportation. Each platoon consists of a platoon headquarters and two sections.

Each platoon headquarters consists of one officer who is the platoon leader and one staff sergeant who is the platoon sergeant.

Each *ambulance section* (2) consists of a sergeant who is the section leader and twelve privates first class or privates. The section is the basic operating unit and operates five motor ambulances.

Equipment and supply. The equipment for an ambulance company is prescribed by Tables of Basic Allowances and by Tables of Equipment.

Supplies are obtained by formal or informal requisition on the regimental supply officer and are drawn by company personnel and transport at the regimental distributing point for such supplies, or they are delivered to the ambulance station by the headquarters and service company of the medical regiment.

The *transportation* of the ambulance company consists of:

    1 truck, ½-ton, command
    1 truck, ½-ton, pick-up
    1 truck, 1½-ton, cargo
    1 truck, 1½-ton cargo, with winch
    1 trailer, 1-ton, cargo
    1 trailer, tank, water, 250-gallon
    1 motorcycle, with side car
   20 ambulances, field, cross-country (five
       ambulances per section)

The primary American-made ambulance was a converted Dodge truck. Called a "Half-tonner," it had a six cylinder engine rated at eighty-five brake horsepower and four forward speeds. It measured sixteen feet three inches long and six feet four inches wide in ambulance form. Under the Lend-Lease program, this vehicle was supplied to other nations.

An ambulance specifically intended for front line work was the Rover 9. Built in Great Britain, the bodywork was entirely aluminum with thermal insulation. It offered room for two stretchers or one stretcher and three seated wounded or six seated wounded.

The Bedford ambulance was widely used on all fronts during WWII, and it was supplied to most of the Allied nations, including America. This ambulance could carry four stretchers, two each side, or ten seated wounded. It was nineteen feet long, nine feet two inches high, and seven feet three inches wide. It had a seventy-two brake horsepower engine. Some vehicles of this type were used by the Civil Defense organization in Great Britain.

Half-track configurations adapted well for ambulance duty, especially in the rescue of airmen whose aircraft were damaged and came down in the sea enroute to their base. They were well suited for operation on the beaches and dunes of Holland and France. Operated by the Coast Guard, these vehicles patrolled the coast with a rescue crew, medical stores, and dinghies. The spotter plane, a Fieseler Storch, was also used in the rescue work.

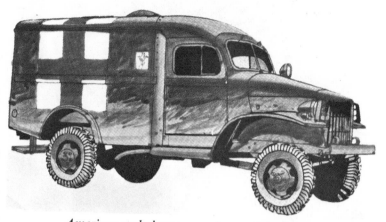

American ambulance manufactured by Dodge.

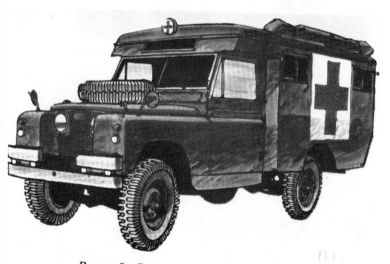

Rover 9, British front line ambulance.

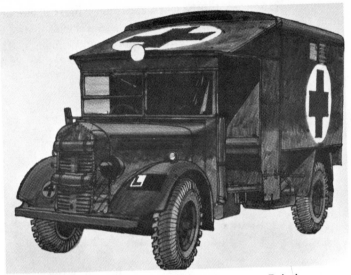

Bedford ambulance made in Great Britain.

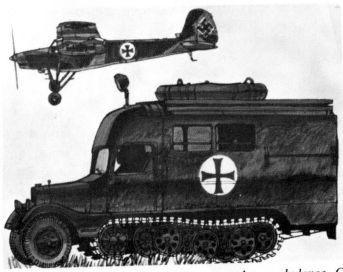

Leichte Zugkraftwagen Sd Kfz 11 converted to ambulance, Germany. (From Ellis, C., Military Transport of World War II, Macmillan Company, 1971)

The following pages illustrate the methods used in the transportation of the sick and wounded as found in the United States *Military Medical Manual.*

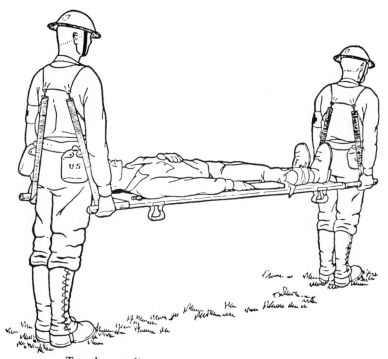

Two-bearer litter squad carrying wounded.

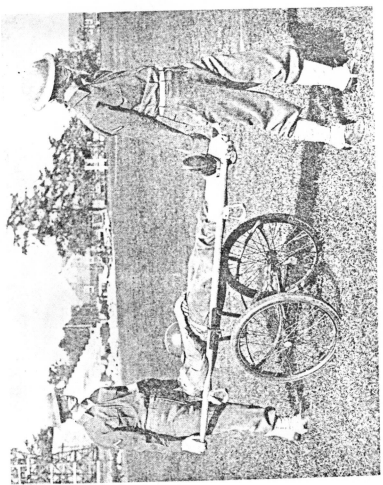

The wheeled litter carrier.

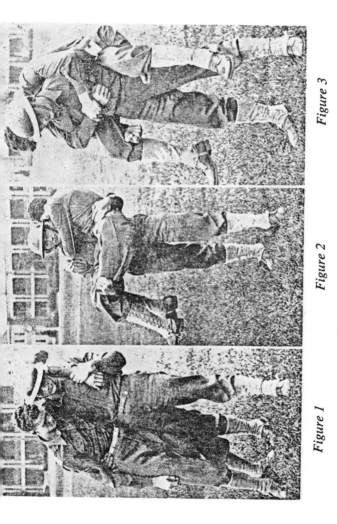

Figure 1   *Figure 2*   *Figure 3*

Pictured above are three means of manual transport of wounded by one-man carry. The method shown in Figure 1 is called the "supporting carry." Figure 2 illustrates the "arms carry," and Figure 3 the "straddle-back carry."

125

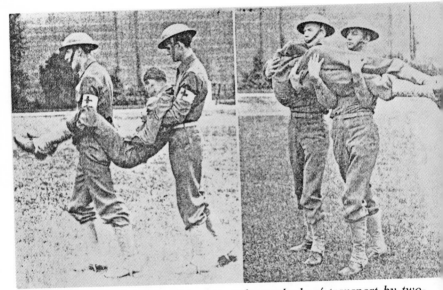

Shown in these two pictures are the methods of transport by two-bearers. The photo on the left illustrates the "saddle-back carry," and the photo on the right shows a wounded man being transported by the "arms carry."

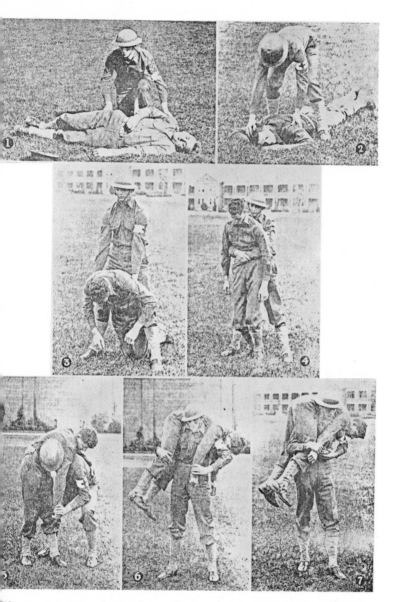

The seven steps shown here illustrate the method of transport known as the "fireman's carry."

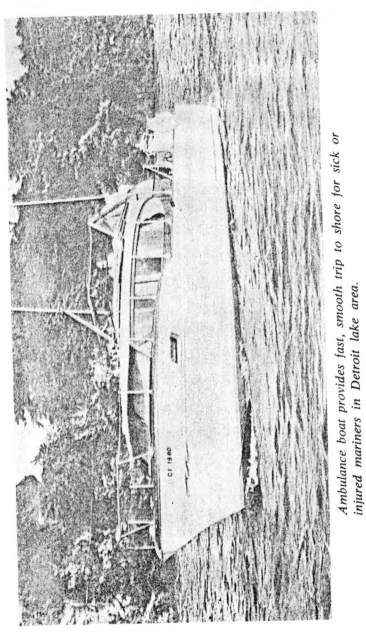

Ambulance boat provides fast, smooth trip to shore for sick or injured mariners in Detroit lake area.

12

Post-World War II Advances in Ambulance Service

THE AMBULANCE BOAT
GREAT LAKES—1961

The first ambulance boat in the Detroit lake area was operated by the Superior Ambulance Company. Walter Gutowski, owner of the company, saw the need for a water ambulance, when he discovered that tugs and barges transported sick and wounded from ship to shore.

He knew it was important to get oxygen and other life saving equipment to the victim immediately. The marine ambulance can keep in touch with the ship by two-way marine radio. It is a thirty-one-foot express cruiser, equipped with portable resuscitator, stretchers, splints, skin diving gear, and all first aid facilities.

The Humphrey Morris—1962

The Corporation of London Port Health Authority put the *Humphrey Morris* into service in 1962 in the Thames estuary to carry out errands of mercy to ships of all nationalities. The ship acts as an ambulance launch, transporting patients from incoming boats to shore for hospitalization. The craft is equipped to care for the patient in hospital-like facilities during the period of transportation. The *Howard Deighton* served for twenty-nine years in this capacity.

Star of Life I—1976

In 1976, the *Star of Life I,* a thirty-one-foot Uniflite cruiser with emergency medical equipment was based in Stamford, Connecticut. Operated under the direction of the Coast Guard and area Marina Police, it provides free medical emergency rescue and patrol duty on Long Island Sound from Norwalk to Greenwich, Connecticut. Owned by Fairfield Medical Products Corporation of Stamford, the boat is staffed by volunteers who, so far, have donated 1,480 hours of their time. The crew consists of doctors, nurses, and emergency medical technicians from the Stamford Ambulance Corps, Stamford Marina Police, and U.S. Coast Guard Auxiliary. The *Star of Life I* is on stand-by duty during the week and is on patrol duty on weekends and holidays. For medical emergencies, help can be requested over marine radio channel 16 or channel 9 on CB radios.

The *Star of Life I* has assisted in many emergencies. Only twenty-seven persons needed more extensive medical help. It has been credited with saving several lives.

Emergency medical instrumentation in the cabin of the *Star of Life I* ambulance boat provides medical and para-medical

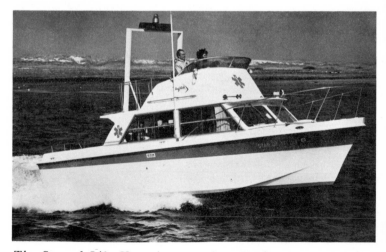

The Star of Life II, *a forty-two-foot Uniflite, was taken into service on December 6, 1976. She operates out of St. John, U.S. Virgin Islands. (Courtesy of Ernst Schindele, President of Fairfield Medical Products)*

personnel with the equipment to start vital life-saving medical care the moment the victim is brought aboard for transport ashore to a hospital. Mounted on the Fairfield Rail across the window above the patient are (left to right): pulse tachometer with photoelectric pulse pick-up; aneroid sphygmomanometer (blood pressure monitor); stop clock; otoscope for eye and ear examination; suction jar and high suction unit; I.V. pole and hanger; and oxygen flowmeter with nebulizer. These instruments are quickly interchangeable or may be easily removed with a flick of the snap-lock that holds them to the rail. On the shelf at the patient's head are (left to right): auxiliary ECG monitoring scope; the Fairfield Combi scope and recorder for coronary surveillance; and the Fairfield Cardio-Aid portable defibrillator. A manual resuscitator is placed over the mouth of the "patient," a Laerdal Resusci-Anne medical training mannikin. Electrodes can be seen connected to the patient's wrists, ankles, and chest. (See picture below.)

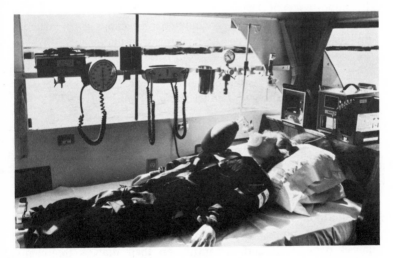

MEDICOPTER

Helicopter evacuation of men wounded in combat in Korea and Vietnam with emergency care before and during flight to the hospital has shown that the helicopter can be a major factor in saving lives.

The Ohio Army National Guard, the highway patrol, and the University hospitals cooperate to save lives in Ohio. A National Guard UH-19D helicopter has been adapted for emergency use and is based in Columbus, Ohio.

The helicopter has walk-around space for two or three medical workers and room for two stretchers and medical equipment. A longitudinal pole with hooks is placed along the ceiling to hold bottles for intravenous fluid administration.

Lessons learned after experimenting with the use of the Medicopter were: (1) The need for an integrated team effort; (2) The importance of keeping intravenous fluids warm; (3) The need to change state laws so qualified physician's assistants may administer fluids and drugs and perform intubations.

The Johnstown, Pennsylvania, Flood of 1977

When the night of July 19, 1977, brought on a Johnstown flood once again, the helicopter was a priceless asset, not only for flying the injured to hospitals outside of the flooded area but also to bring in medical supplies. Medication as well as food supplies were in dire need of refrigeration. The helicopters brought in ice. Blood supplies were rendered useless during the power outage. New blood was flown in by helicopter. Some thirty dialysis patients dependent for life on their dialysis treatments, were flown to Pittsburgh Presbyterian Hospital for their lifesaving therapy.

The valley would have been completely isolated if it had not been for the helicopter. It is truly a RESCUE vehicle.

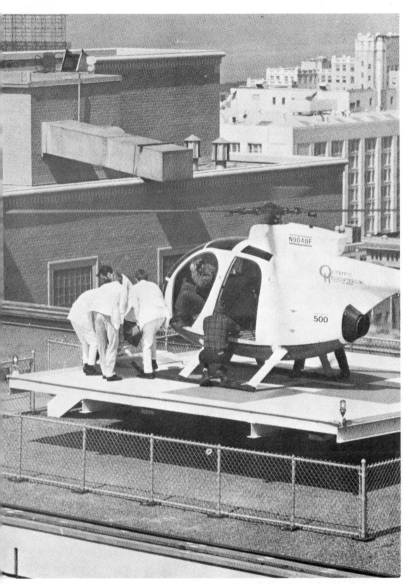

The medicopter crew in operation at Virginia Mason Hospital, Seattle, Washington. (Courtesy of Perspective, *the Blue Cross and Blue Shield magazine)*

133

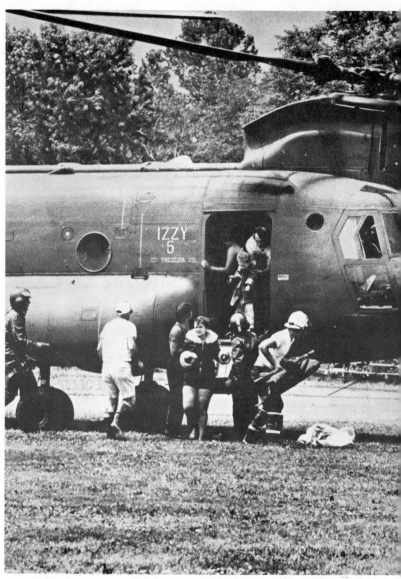

Helicopter in use during the Johnstown Flood of 1977. (Courtesy of Tribune-Review, *Greensburg, Pennsylvania)*

THE AMBULANCE AND ITS ROLE
IN THE EARLY CORONARY CARE SYSTEM

Approximately six hundred thousand Americans die of heart attack every year. But more tragic is the fact that more than half of all heart-attack deaths occur before the victim is reached by medical treatment of any kind. Records further show that fifty to sixty percent of all heart-attack deaths occur within the first hour following the attack.

Many of these deaths can be prevented by Early Coronary Care, mainly through defibrillation. In the opinion of Dr. William J. Grace of Saint Vincent's Hospital, New York City, if defibrillation can be achieved soon enough, ". . . we should lose nobody from ventricular fibrillation in the present day" (from "The Mobile Coronary Care Unit and the Intermediate Coronary Care Unit in the Total Systems Approach to Coronary Care," *Chest*, 1970).

As summarized in an article by Dr. Stuart Bondurant, "The pre-hospital phase of acute myocardial infarction poses the greatest single medical problem of our nation in terms of loss of potentially salvageable life."

What is an Early Coronary Care System?

An Early Coronary Care System provides for treatment of the cardiac emergency patient prior to his admission to coronary care facilities in the hospital. Ideally, such a system will consist of sophisticated communications networks, speeded-up reception procedures at hospital cardiac centers, and mobile coronary care units in specially equipped vehicles.

Basically, Early Coronary Care Systems act to bring the thoroughly trained personnel and basic equipment of the in-hospital coronary care unit to the patient as quickly as possible.

The American Heart Association lists the following as the early warning signs of heart attack. Prolonged, oppressive pain or unusual discomfort in the center of chest, behind the breastbone. Pain may radiate to the shoulder, arm, neck or jaw. The pain or discomfort is often accompanied by sweating; nausea, vomiting, and shortness of breath may also occur. Sometimes these symptoms subside and then return.

Minutes count when heart attack strikes. Act promptly. Call a doctor and carefully describe the symptoms. If no doctor is immediately available, get the victim to a hospital emergency room at once.

FIRST MOBILE CORONARY UNIT
AND "FLYING SQUAD"

For two years prior to 1966, organized resuscitation methods were applied in the treatment of cardiac arrest at the Royal Victoria Hospital, Belfast, Ireland. In thirty out of sixty-three patients, resuscitation was successful. Where arrest occurred in a general medical ward or in the casualty department, there were thirteen long-term survivors, or thirty-one percent.

It was this fact of thirty-one percent survival of patients not in the intensive-care area which gave Dr. Pantridge the idea that if the same kind of resuscitation team could "reach the patient in his home immediately after the occurrence of coronary occlusion, a considerable reduction in the mortality might be achieved."

Portable Heart Shocker

Dr. J. F. Pantridge has now developed a defibrillator or heart-shocker which is capable of administering electric shock to the chest through the metal paddles to restore normal heartbeat which has been stopped or disturbed by a heart attack.

The first heart-shockers which were portable weighed more than one hundred pounds. They were awkward and cumbersome. The new one weighs less than eight pounds and is powered by batteries. Dr. Pantridge suggests that the defibrillator should be in each doctor's office, at sports events and wherever there is a crowd situation.

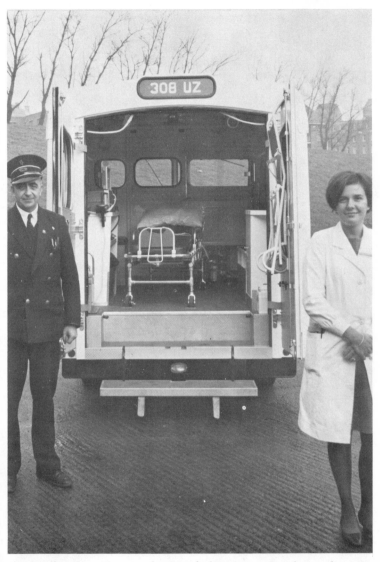

An inside view of a modern ambulance as seen from the rear.
(Courtesy of Dr. J. F. Pantridge, photographs by Robert J.
Anderson & Co., Belfast, Ireland)

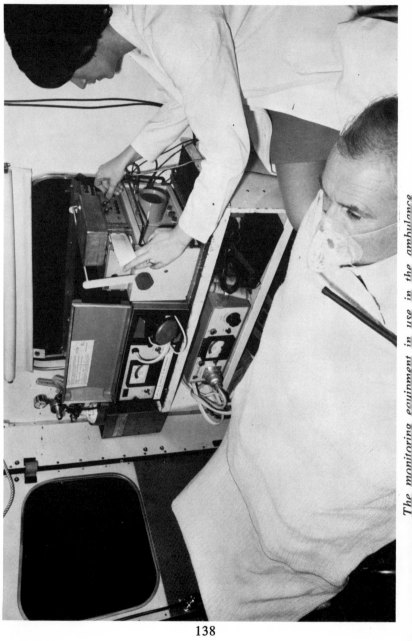

The monitoring equipment in use in the ambulance

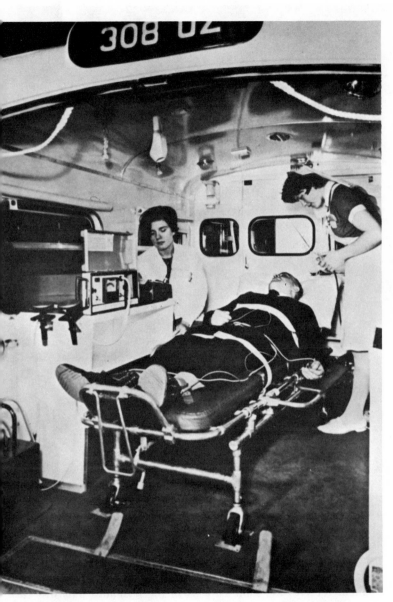

A patient in transport in a mobile coronary care unit.

139

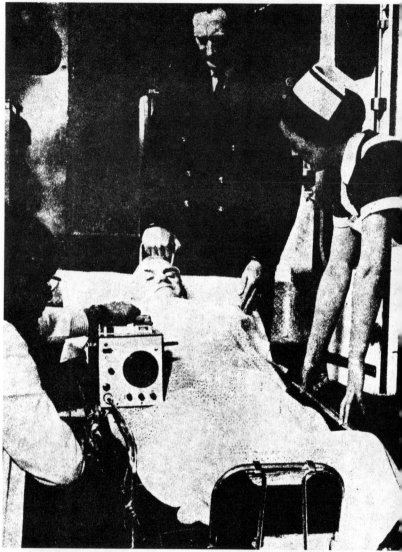

A patient is shown being moved from the ambulance to the coronary care unit of a hospital. While in the ambulance the patient receives the same care as in the hospital's intensive care unit.

140

THE HEARTMOBILE

It is a well-known fact that most deaths from myocardial infarction occur before the patient can be admitted to the hospital. Use of a mobile coronary unit would therefore improve greatly the chances of survival. The cost, both initial and operational, of maintaining a "heart ambulance" is prohibitive to most communities.

However, in San Francisco, California, a system has been found which is fairly efficient. Mount Zion Hospital in cooperation with Electro-Biometrics of Lancaster, California, and the San Francisco Ambulance Service, a private ambulance company, are providing a valuable service to heart disease patients.

The operation of the telemetry system occurs as follows. The physician calls the ambulance company and instructs it to take the patient to the hospital and monitor the patient. When the ambulance attendants arrive and take the patient into the ambulance, disposable ECG electrodes are taped to the chest. The attendants radio the ambulance base dispatcher who then telephones the hospital coronary care unit. The demodulator and tape recorder are turned on in the coronary care unit. The ambulance dispatcher connects the phone patch which permits the hospital personnel to speak directly to the ambulance. Data transmission and voice communication use the same line, the sound of the voice automatically shutting off the data transmission. Under these circumstances the telemetry serves to put the physician's skills in the ambulance with the trained ambulance attendant acting as his hands.

The concept of a mobile coronary unit developed from the pioneering work of Dr. J. F. Pantridge in Belfast, Ireland, where a unit was first used in January, 1966.

Many communities are now finding it justifiable to establish mobile coronary units because so many lives can be saved by this service.

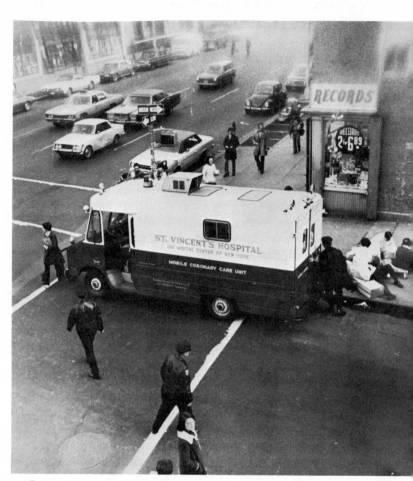

Saint Vincent's MCCU, initiated in 1968, was the first such vehicle to be used in New York. Fully fitted with cardiac equipment and staffed with physicians, the MCCU brings hospital-quality care directly to the patient within a matter of minutes, providing heart attack victims with a seventy-five percent chance of survival during their first hour of attack.
(Courtesy of Saint Vincent's Hospital and Medical Center, New York)

142

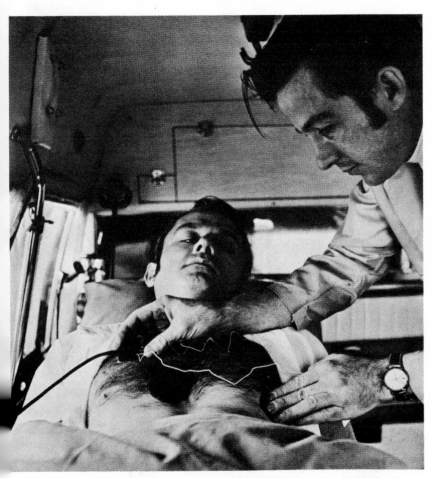

The heartmobile in action. Voice communication is established with the hospital coronary care unit on the same line on which the ECG is transmitted.

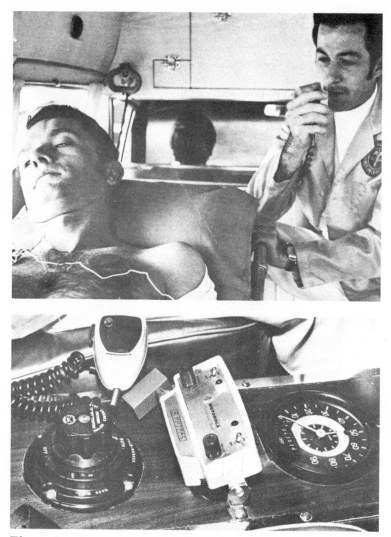

The patient is reassured, and the ambulance attendant is guided by hearing the voice of a physician. When not used for voice communications the line becomes free for relaying the modulator ECG signals by powerful radio transmitter back to ambulance headquarters. (Photos courtesy of Hess and Eisenhardt Company)

144

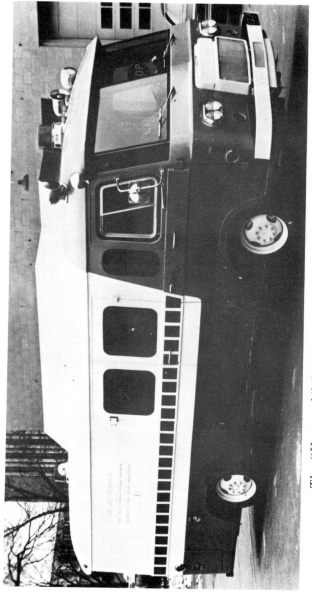

The "Heartmobile"—Department of Medicine, Ohio State University, Columbus, Ohio, Dave Ellies Industrial Design, Inc. (Courtesy of Dr. James V. Warren)

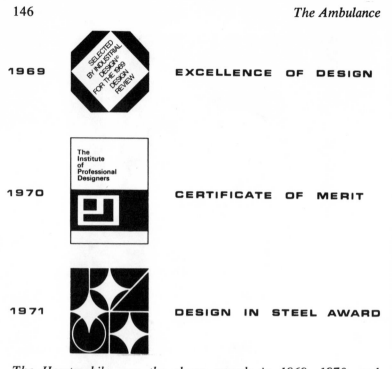

1969		EXCELLENCE OF DESIGN
1970		CERTIFICATE OF MERIT
1971		DESIGN IN STEEL AWARD

The Heartmobile won the above awards in 1969, 1970, and 1971.

THE COLUMBUS STORY
OF MOBILE EMERGENCY MEDICAL CARE

BY

JAMES V. WARREN, M.D.
Chairman Department of Medicine
Ohio State University College of Medicine

A medical emergency may happen to anyone, anytime, anywhere. From that moment on, the care the victims receive has a direct bearing on their return to health. This begins with

Mobile Emergency Medical Care—a program which was founded in Columbus, Ohio, and has made significant progress in the last seven years. Not only has this resulted in greatly improved patient care, but new capabilities have been acquired and new abilities have been mastered as well.

The Columbus Ohio Division of Fire was one of the first departments in the United States to offer a Mobile Emergency Medical Care service to the public beginning in 1934. Columbus's efforts reflect the growth of Emergency Medical Care in the United States.

Each year fifty million people experience a medical emergency outside the hospital. Documented research shows that a significant reduction in mortality is realized by effective and efficient emergency medical care. This care can be achieved in communities where the will to provide it exists.

Columbus Fire-Fighters Pioneer Emergency Care

Fire fighting has always been one of the most hazardous occupations in the country. As a result, it was not uncommon to find a physician at the scene of a major fire drawn there both by the need for professional services and the "fire buff's" thrill of following the "engines." Historically, many volunteer fire companies listed physicians on their membership rosters.

In the period following World War I and as motorized fire apparatus came into service, fire departments in major cities added an ambulance to their equipment roster and first aid kits to the rigs. This care capability was provided for the fire fighters and civilian victims of the emergency.

In 1931 a Lyons pulmotor was donated to the Columbus Fire Department and was carried in the chief's buggy for the protection of fire fighters overcome by smoke. In 1933, Chief Edward Welch recommended the formation of an emergency squad in his first annual report; however, the event that effected the birth of a squad service was the electrocution of a lineman working on a pole in 1934. Chief Welch responded to the call for help with two fire fighters and the pulmotor. Although attempts to save the lineman was futile, newspaper coverage of the fire department's efforts resulted in citizens calling the fire department for aid in a medical emergency. Late in 1934, a hose wagon equipped with supplies donated by the Red Cross along with an H and H Inhalator was placed in service for the public; thus Columbus Fire Department became one of the first fire departments in the country to offer this service.

From that date in 1934, "Number One Inhalator" steadily gained the support of the citizenry and the medical community. Each year more requests for aid came, additional squads were placed into service, and more men were trained. The squadmen developed a sincere interest in their work, attending classes on their own time and practicing their skills under the supervision of physicians who volunteered their services. Patient care improved and first aid teams were formed. The Columbus teams have demonstrated their ability by placing in the top ten positions in the International Rescue and First Aid competitions since 1963.

National Attention Focuses on Effectiveness

In the early 1960s Emergency Medical Care began to receive national attention. The long-range implications of efficient and effective emergency medical care on mortality were pointed out in a report by the National Research Council, National Science Foundation, entitled "Accidental Death and Disability, the Neglected Disease of Modern Society." Columbus had a highly trained fire department Emergency Squad which arrived at the scene on an average of four minutes after a call for help. Yet nationally, mobile emergency medical teams arrived at an average response time of over forty minutes with inadequately equipped and trained crews. Primarily as a result of concern over highway safety, specifications were developed at a national level covering ambulance attendant training and equipment requirements as well as the design of the emergency vehicle itself.

A major new concern of the medical community at this time

was heart attacks. As the number one cause of death in the United States, heart attacks were claiming close to a million lives a year. Technical developments leading to knowledge about alarm systems, electrical defibrillation, and closed chest pulmonary resuscitation, resulted in the formation of Coronary Care Units (CCU) in major hospitals. The Ohio State University Hospitals opened the first Coronary Care Unit in Columbus in 1964.

While positive studies could now be made toward reducing the death rate of patients who reached the CCU, any major reduction in the overall mortality rate was still limited because of the incidence of "sudden death" before the victim reached the CCU.

In 1966 Dr. J. F. Pantridge proposed the use of "flying squads" to provide pre-hospital care to coronary disease victims in Belfast, Northern Ireland. These special coronary care vehicles would go out with a physician to treat heart attack victims at the scene. Their ability to stabilize the vicitm at the scene prior to transporting him had dramatic results and aroused interest in the U.S.A.

In 1965, the Armco Steel Corporation sponsored their first annual Student Design Program. One student teacher from the University of Cincinnati analyzed the then traditional ambulance. Their design efforts served as the catalyst which stimulated the idea of a Mobile Coronary Care Van.

Heartmobile Concept Founded in Columbus

Research in the concept of mobile emergency care began in Columbus in 1966, and the turning point for emergency care came three years later when the "Heartmobile" became operational. It was the first vehicle of its kind in the United States specifically designed to transport the care and facilities of the CCU directly to the victim. The vehicle was operated in conjunction with the Columbus Fire Department Emergency Squads and financed by a grant from the Regional Medical Program to Ohio State University.

The heartmobile was staffed by three off-duty squadmen and a physician from the Ohio State University Hospitals. The program was an investigational study to determine the merits of mobile emergency coronary care. The results were highly successful.

The outgrowth of this program has been greatly improved emergency service for people in the Columbus metropolitan area. The heartmobile concept was incorporated July 1, 1971 into the pre-existing Fire Rescue Squad system. Experience proved that physician attendance was not necessary. Properly trained squadmen could perform diagnosis and therapy of cardio-vascular emergencies as effectively as physicians. The "medic" units operated in conjunction with standard rescue squads. Seven contiguous communities in conjunction with Columbus dispatch the nearest of thirteen medics and thirty-two emergency squads to the emergency without regard of municipal boundaries.

This system is a forerunner in the country. Fifty-five percent of all heart attacks within the City of Columbus are first seen by medics. The units reach the scene of a medical emergency at an average response time of 3.55 minutes. In Columbus alone fifteen to twenty life-saving rescues are performed each month and more in the suburban areas.

Emergency medicine, effectively practiced from the call for help until the victim is placed in the care of a physician, can have a dramatic effect on mortality. The goal now is to bring this level of patient care to as many people as possible in a practical and economical manner.

Undoubtedly, the emergency operations of the Columbus Division of Fire and the Fire Service as a whole will continue to develop and, as medical knowledge and facilities increase, so will that of the Mobile Emergency Medical team. The proposed ambulance of the future, which is being studied in Columbus, and the widening array of techniques available to emergency medical teams will increase the scope of their activity and provide the best emergency medical care. It is anticipated that this will be coupled with increasing sophistication of the hospital emergency facilities and will also be incorporated into a central operation of emergency vehicles within an appropriate call and response system.

Mobile Emergency Medical Care has made great progress in the last five years. The skills and procedures practiced by the Mobile Medical team have increased in scope and complexity with a direct and positive benefit to the victim. The challenge of today will be its growth in the next five years.

RESCUE 52, CINCINNATI, OHIO, PARAMEDICS—1973

Of more than six hundred thousand deaths from heart attacks expected in the United States during 1973, more than half would occur during the first hour after the onset of the episode.

It was the goal of Rescue 52 to train paramedics to take the appropriate expertise and equipment to the patient. Stabilization of his vital signs would then be accomplished before his trip to the hospital where continued, less frantic treatment could be carried on.

The steering committee for "52" was comprised of representatives from the Academy of Medicine, University of Cincinnati Medical Center, American Heart Association Southwestern Ohio Chapter, Hamilton County Disaster Council, Cincinnati Fire Department, City and County communications Centers, Hamilton County Chapter of the American Red Cross, The Health Planning Association of the Central Ohio River Valley, the Cincinnati Association of Life Underwriters, and Merrell-National Laboratories. Dr. Robert McMaster of Merrell-National was chairman of the project.

The name *Rescue 52* was chosen to honor the original Cincinnati Fire Department life squad unit, Squad 52.

This project is now completed and the maintenance of ambulance equipment and paramedic training has been assumed by the city.

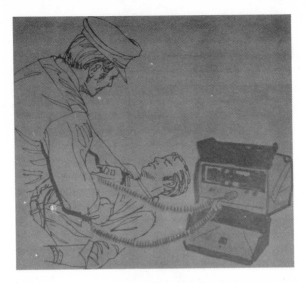

Rescue 52

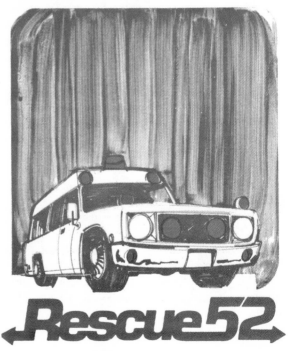

ACT FOUNDATION

The acronym ACT stands for "Advanced Coronary Treatment." It is a non-profit group consisting of nine pharmaceutical firms founded to stimulate physician and public interest in improving emergency care systems nationwide.

For an emergency system to succeed, many groups in the community must be involved, as well as city and county officials, firemen and police, medical institutions, and industry. The Foundation's job is to inform these groups as to practical application and to inspire action. In other words its purposes are educational and motivational. ACT does not grant funds.

The Foundation concentrates on coronary treatment because this is where the most dramatic results can be obtained. If you have a well equipped mobile coronary unit, the vehicle is equipped to handle most any kind of emergency.

The next emphasis of ACT will be to educate the patient to recognize the symptoms of heart attack so as not to delay calling for emergency care.

Emergency Services: What They Are (*from the* Digest of Surveys)

WHAT DOES AN AMBULANCE CARRY?
Oxygen unit—87%
Resuscitation airways—62%
Bag-mask resuscitator—46%
Oropharyngeal airway—44%
Suction apparatus—43%
Sterile gauze—81%
Adhesive tape—77%
Triangular bandages—70%
Universal dressing—54%
Splints (wood-metal-plastic)—65%
Padded leg splints—42%
Padded arm splints—41%
Half-ring splints—33%
Backboards—30%

WHO OWNS THE AMBULANCES?
Funeral homes—44%
Volunteer groups—24%
Commercial firms—14%
Local government (police and fire depts.)—13%
Hospital-operated—3%
Other—2%

WHAT IS AN AMBULANCE?
Conventional ambulances—36%
Station wagons—24%
Hearses—21%
Panel truck—10%
Rescue vehicles—9%

HOW ARE HOSPITAL
EMERGENCY DEPARTMENTS
RUN?

Twenty-four hour coverage by
   physician—17%
Director a physician—46%
Emergency department
   committee—39%
Written medical-surgical
   procedures—42%
Communitywide hospital disaster
   plan—49%
Individual hospital disaster
   plan—79%
   (Two fifths of this group had a
   trial run within the past year)

WHAT CAN AMBULANCE
ATTENDANTS DO?

Administer oxygen and maintain
   airways—81%
Dress open wounds—80%
Control hemorrhaging—75%
Splint fractures—74%
Care for Burns—64%
Handle emergency births—50%
Cardiac compression—50%
Treat poisoning—39%

THE BABY AMBULANCE—1969

Dr. George L. Baker, assistant professor of pediatrics in the
University of Iowa College of Medicine and director of the Iowa
Infant Study of the State Services for Crippled Children, said
that a standard ambulance does not have enough room for the
equipment and personnel needed to care for a critically ill infant.
Therefore, in 1969, the SSCC and the University of Iowa Health
Center developed a special van, the first designed exclusively
for babies.

The ambulance system serves an area within a ninety-mile
radius of Iowa City. University Hospital in Iowa City is the only
large medical center in the state and the only one equipped to
care for the newborn who is in distress. Babies are transported
from small community hospitals to the University of Iowa Health
Center. The baby van is especially useful for infants requiring
cardiac evaluation, surgery, and respiratory support. Equipment
includes two incubators, oxygen, suction aspirator, heart monitor,
drugs, other supplies, and a two-way radio. The initial cost,

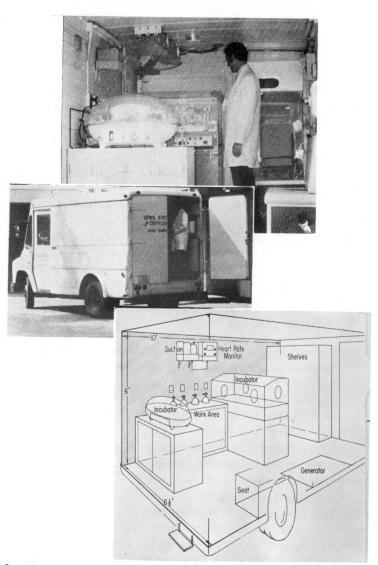

Interior and exterior views of a Sick Baby Van. The diagram on the right is a blueprint of the equipment and working space inside the ambulance. (Journal of the American Medical Association 209, 1969, p. 1826)

including equipment was twelve thousand, six hundred dollars; operating cost is about seventy cents per mile. Helicopter service is also available from distant parts of the state.

The Children's Hospital in Cincinnati, Ohio is also fortunate to have a "Newborn Special Care Unit." Babies who are in need of this special care must be transported to this unit from other hospitals. A specially designed transport incubator accompanied by a physician in an ambulance is the beginning of recovery for many desperately ill children. The doctor can adjust the temperature of the incubator, regulate the humidity and oxygen content of the air, and watch the baby's heart and breathing with special monitoring equipment. Without these special "baby" ambulances, many would die en route to their special care.

The Virginia Polytechnic Institute, Blackburg, Virginia, in cooperation with the Roanoke Memorial Hospital, Roanoke, Virginia, have developed a high-speed transport system for newborns in distress. A twin-engine airplane is equipped with an infant respirator and special incubator. A ground ambulance brings the baby to the airport, the crew transfers the child to the plane and upon arrival, the incubator is again placed in a specially prepared ambulance to be taken to the "Special Care Unit."

A GOLF COURSE RESCUE VEHICLE

After a member of the Rhode Island Country Club had a fatal heart attack on the golf course, members decided to invest in an emergency rescue system.

A converted dune buggy was equipped with life-saving equipment and attendants were trained to use the first aid kit, blankets, and resuscitator. Travel time from the clubhouse to the ninth tee, the farthest on the course, is two and a half minutes.

Air horns are placed in each golf bag as the players go out on the course. Members are being trained to give immediate resuscitation until the dune buggy arrives. They have agreed that ten dollars per member is a small price to pay to save one life. (See page 159.)

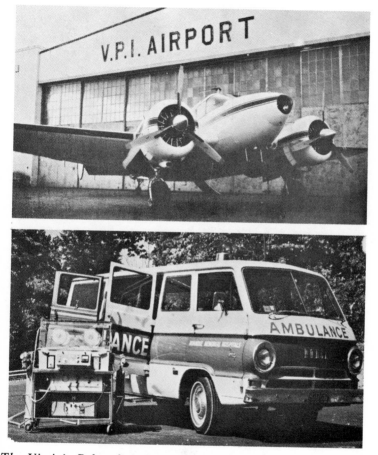

The Virginia Polytechnic Institute airplane is used for the transportation of infants requiring emergency medical care. The ambulance pictured is part of the transport system to and from the airport.

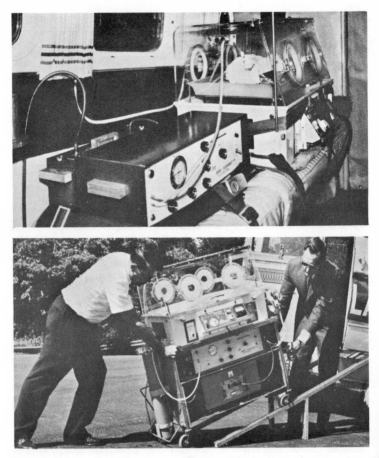

Interior view showing the ARP Respirator and the Armstrong Servo-Control Incubator. As can be seen, respiratory support continues uninterrupted throughout transfer. (Courtesy of Journal of the American Medical Association)

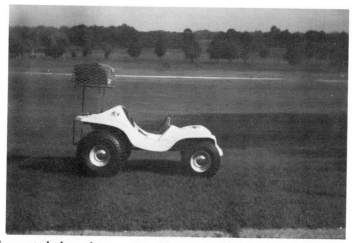

Converted dune buggy with life-saving equipment. (Courtesy of Fred Hulme)

A CAMPUS AMBULANCE SERVICE

Twenty-four hour ambulance service was offered for the first time on the University of Cincinnati campus, a community of fifty-thousand people, in 1971.

One full time employee and seven students were fully trained ambulance attendants. They qualify as Registered Emergency Medical Technicians. In addition to providing service for individual emergencies, the ambulance and squad attend athletic events and are prepared to take care of players or spectators when needed. The life squad offers courses in first aid to students. They inspect first aid kits in dormitories once a month.

In November, 1972 an unknown donor gave nine-thousand dollars for the purchase of a new ambulance. It is fully equipped with a built-in oxygen system, a pulse tachometer, light rescue equipment, and a hydraulic jack that can separate or lift vehicles involved in an accident.

Before the ambulance came to the campus, a station wagon was used. At that time ambulance runs increased from 1,469 in 1968 to 2,109 runs in 1969 and 4,191 in 1972.

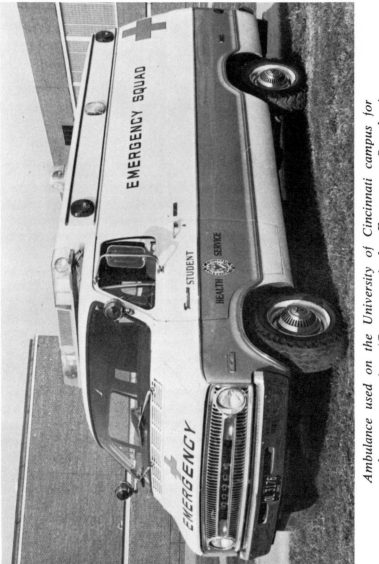

Ambulance used on the University of Cincinnati campus for student emergencies. (Courtesy of the Emergency Squad of University of Cincinnati, Ohio)

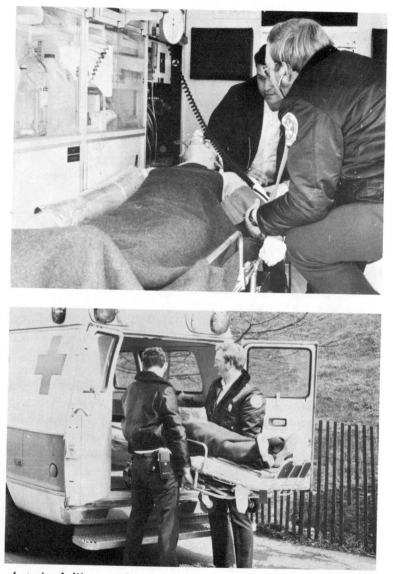

A trained life squad on the University of Cincinnati campus administers emergency treatment. (Courtesy of Emergency Squad, University of Cincinnati)

13

Continuing Programs
for the Improvement
of Ambulance Service

COMMITTEE ON TRAUMA RESPONSIBLE FOR
IMPROVED SERVICE IN EMERGENCIES

The committee on Trauma of the American College of Surgeons was established in 1922. Although the name has been changed several times, the original objective has been unchanged—*improvement in the care of the injured*. Regional committees, state/provincial, and local have been active. There are fifty-eight state committees. Several major metropolitan areas have been given status because of the large population represented. All but one of these committees have projects under way designed to improve ambulance service. Their voices were usually unheard by local government officials. When the National Highway Safety Bureau was created, the Trauma Committees were there to promote the use of federal funds.

In 1957, the Trauma Committee of the American Association for the Surgery of Trauma and the National Safety Council formed a joint Action Program which sponsored a nationwide survey of emergency services.

Three grants from the John A. Hartford Foundation established the Trauma Field Program with Dr. Robert Kennedy as the Director. The survey of ambulance equipment and service shocked those who read the results. Almost immediately, the committee developed a list of "Minimum Equipment for Ambulances." The list was updated in 1969 by Dr. J. D. Farrington. *Essential Equipment for Ambulances* is now the nationally accepted standard. In 1970, Dr. Farrington published a *Curriculum for Training for Emergency Medical Technicians—Ambulance*. Dr. Kennedy has been the leader in promoting and providing educational materials on emergency care and services for the last decade.

PARAMEDIC BEGINNINGS

Dr. Peter Safar of the University Health Center of Pittsburgh is one of the leading figures in the concern for improvement in ambulance services. When "Emergency" comes on television everyone is thrilled and excited with the excellence of the paramedic's performance. Unfortunately many communities do not have the TV type of emergency care. Dr. Safar has been promoting the training of ambulance attendants in Pittsburgh for many years. He is an anesthesiologist especially concerned with resuscitation in emergency situations. In 1967 he started a unique project called Freedom House Ambulance Service. With the help of a group of concerned citizens who were encouraging Black enterprise, forty people were picked out of the ghetto. They were enrolled in a class for three hundred hours of classroom work followed by nine months of physician supervised work on the ambulances. Clinical experience was found by the students in operating rooms, intensive care units, and emergency rooms. In 1968, Freedom House Ambulance started a service with the city which gave prehospital care and saved lives to such a remarkable extent that Pittsburgh was overwhelmed.

Dr. Safar suggested expanding the service and improving ambulance vehicles. But here the success story stopped because the grant-type funding ran out and the city was too "broke" to maintain the services. In 1966, Governor Lawrence had died in a police ambulance but the tragedy did not lead to upgrading ambulance service.

The same pattern is true in many other cities and communities where grants and private funding stopped and municipal gov-

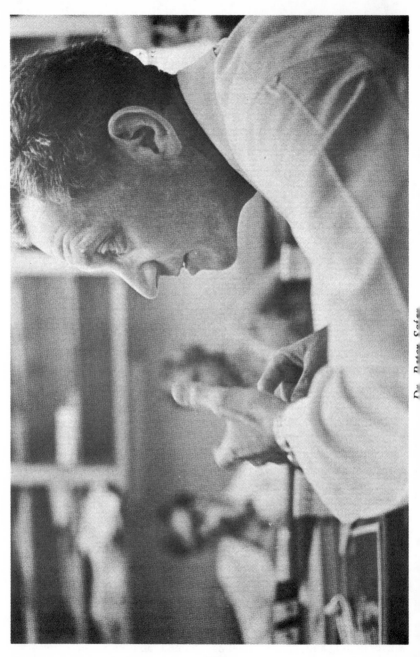

Dr. Peter Safar

ernments were not able to finance the continued ambulance service.

It was one of Dr. Safar's dreams to standardize paramedic training. In January, 1975, the President's Interagency Committee on Emergency Medical Service recommended that a standard curriculum be developed. In July, 1975, the United States Department of Transportation (USDOT) announced a plan made up of three basic parts: a course guide, instructor lesson plans, and a student study guide. This represented the first step towards national standardization of paramedic training.

In 1966 ambulance service usually consisted of transportation in the back of a police paddy wagon, madly racing to the hospital. There were practically no trained ambulance attendants. The patient lived in spite of the ambulance ride. By 1977, there were some eight to ten thousand paramedics and thousands of lives had been saved because of their dedication. What a tragedy is in store if communities do not become concerned enough to carry on the support of updated ambulance services!

AMBULANCE ATTENDANTS (EMTs) TRAINING PROGRAMS*

A. *Level I:* 70-100 hours (depending on type of teacher and backgrounds of trainees)

   1. Equivalent of American Red Cross Standard and Advanced First Aid Course (25 hours)
   2. Anatomy, physiology (5 to 10 hours) including recognition and management of vital system dysfunction
   3. Life-support (12 hours) with manikin practice
      American Heart Association CPR Course
      Airway care, ventilation, oxygenation (including safe handling of compressed gas systems), external cardiac compression to perfection
      Management of serious and life-threatening medical emergencies

---

*(*Courtesy* of Anesthesia and Analgesia . . . Current Researches, *51:28, 29, 1972*)

4. Control of hemorrhage, treatment of shock and wound care (2 hours)
5. Extremity fractures (2 hours)
6. Defensive driving, control at accident scene, emergency vehicle operation, equipment (6 hours)
7. Rescue and release from entrapment including extrication of spine injured patients
8. Co-ordinated disaster response and management of multiple casualties (2 hours)
9. Communications (2 hours)
10. Records, forms, debriefing (2 hours)
11. Obstetrics, childbirth, and newborn resuscitation (2 hours)
12. Pediatrics, neonatal transfer (2 hours)
13. Poisoning and burns (2 hours)
14. Psychiatry (2 hours)
15. Health services organization, hospital relationships, medicolegal aspects (1 hour)
16. Observation in hospital ER, OR, PAR, ICU (10 hours minimum)

B. *Level II:* approximately 3 to 4 months; hospital-based training in addition to Level I training (70 to 100 hours)

1. Clinical rotations coupled with appropriate didactic and seminar sessions (sequence depends upon rotation)
    a. Practice of resuscitation including definitive care technics during transfer
    b. Recovery room (life-support techniques, monitoring, venous infusion)
    c. Cardiac care unit (arrhythmia control)
    d. ICU (life-support techniques, care of intubated and tracheotomized patient)
    e. Emergency room
    f. Inhalation therapy
    g. Delivery room
    h. Morgue (Medical Examiner)

2. Special exercise (may be during rotation of [I])
   a. Practice of resuscitation including definitive care technics during transfer
   b. Practice of light rescue and extrication
   c. Use of definitive care (physician's) equipment at scene and in transit
   d. Training in observation and communication (verbal and written) techniques (code communication, radio usage, report forms, etc)

3. Cardiac care (1 month); arrhythmia recognition and control under physician direction (electrocardiogram, use of drugs, defibrillation, telemetry)
4. On-the-job field experience (additional 1 month)
5. Ambulance service administration and operations

C. *Level III:* 2 to 4 years hospital and college education; university degree

Dr. Peter Safar graduated from the University of Vienna, Austria. He completed his training at Yale Medical School. He has been active in the fields of resuscitation, emergency care, intensive care, and the public health aspects of anesthesiology. He is cofounder and 1972 president of the newly formed multidisciplinary Society of Critical Care Medicine.

REPORT OF THE NATIONAL ACADEMY OF SCIENCES

The National Academy of Sciences, Washington, D.C., reported to the nation that emergency services are "one of the weakest links in the delivery of health care in the nation. . . . Thousands of lives are lost through lack of systematic application of established principles of emergency care."

The American Medical Association has sponsored legislation that asks for a new department of Emergency Medicine in the Department of Health, Education and Welfare. The proposed

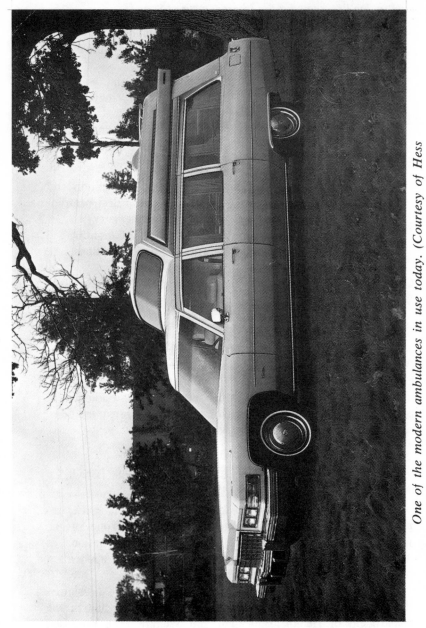

One of the modern ambulances in use today. (Courtesy of Hess and Eisenhardt Company, Cincinnati, Ohio)

168

legislation calls for the upgrading of emergency care by improving the quality of ambulance vehicles and first aid administered by attendants.

The report stated that some one hundred and ten thousand Americans die and eleven million are in bed at least one day each year from accident injuries. The Academy recommends that responsibility for planning and coordination should be based in the Office of the President. Under a national plan, life-saving measures could be taken as follows:

1. Upgrade quality of ambulances to replace 80% of the twenty-five thousand in the country that are hearses, station wagons, and limousines and are inadequately equipped.

2. Establish "911" as the emergency telephone number nationwide.

3. Set up urban and regional emergency communications centers that use radio frequencies. Operators should know medical terminology.

4. Train a nationwide corps of emergency medical technicians to be assigned to ambulances to start immediate care of the patient while en route to the hospital. Only one-third of present attendants have had adequate training.

5. Categorize hospitals according to their abilities and readiness to provide professional care.

6. Hospital emergency rooms should be staffed twenty-four hours a day with qualified physicians. Medical schools should train students in emergency medicine and hospitals should establish more residencies for young doctors interested in this type of practice.

7. Nurses should be trained for immediate care of emergencies.

8. Funds spent for research in trauma or accident care, should be expanded reflecting the fact that accidents are the leading killers of young Americans.

FOUR IMPORTANT BOOKLETS NECESSARY
TO THE DEVELOPMENT OF
ADEQUATE COMMUNITY EMERGENCY SERVICES

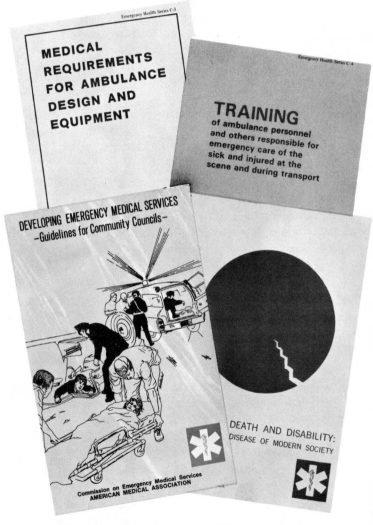

Current editions are available from A.M.A.

14

Ambulance of the Future

This is an artist's drawing of the "Lifemobile," a new proto-type ambulance. It was designed by Frederick M. Hill, president of the Medilogic Design Systems in Columbus, Ohio, and is funded by the Armco Foundation of the Armco Steel Corporation of Middletown, Ohio. The endeavor is being coordinated by the ACT Foundation, a public service group sponsored by twelve leading pharmaceutical companies. ACT, which stands for Advanced Coronary Treatment, has worked for better design in emergency vehicles since its inception in 1969.

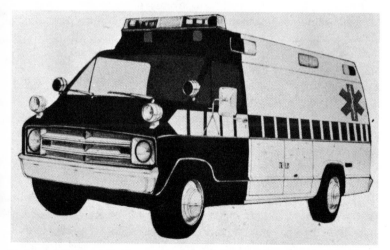

"Lifemobile," ambulance of the future. (Courtesy of Frederick M. Hill)

LIFEMOBILE

The "Lifemobile" was a concept incorporating the best features of the ambulance and the guidelines put forth by emergency medical teams in order to produce a super-efficient, life-saving vehicle. The ACT Foundation and Armco Steel Corporation sponsored a two-year study to devise an effective mobile environment for emergency medical care. The suggestions of the research team became reality with the design of this vehicle named "Lifemobile." Improvements were made in five major areas: patient accessibility, attendant work areas, storage capability, safety, and economics. The primary goal of this program was to improve patient care, and that goal has apparently been reached.

SUPERAMBULANCE

Tomorrow's ambulance will be an emergency room on wheels. It is estimated that at least ten to twenty percent of fatalities of accident victims could be prevented by prompt and adequate first aid at the scene.

The means for giving this immediate service must be provided by expanding and extending the ambulance to include life saving and supporting equipment which the personnel is capable of using. Today's ambulance is too small.

A vehicle of sufficient size and properly equipped could act as an emergency room at the scene as well as a conveyance to the hospital. In case of a major disaster, the superambulance could act as a triage station at the scene while conventional ambulances would transport the prepared patients to the hospital.

Dr. Herbert Warm of Vista, California, a retired U.S. Naval Research Captain has maintained an interest in emergency vehicles since he first rode an ambulance in medical school. He claims the initial problem of the emergency vehicle is the size. The standard ambulance is too small for a medical team to give emergency treatment. He has in mind a Travco 270 executive unit. The twenty-

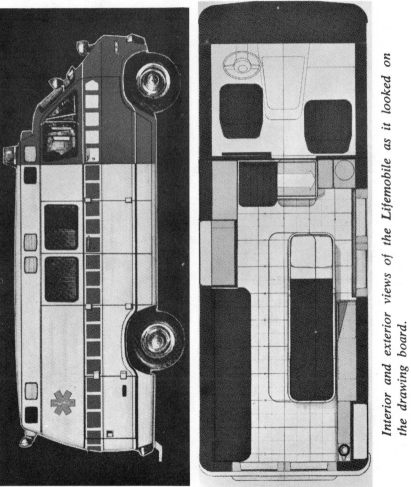

Interior and exterior views of the Lifemobile as it looked on the drawing board.

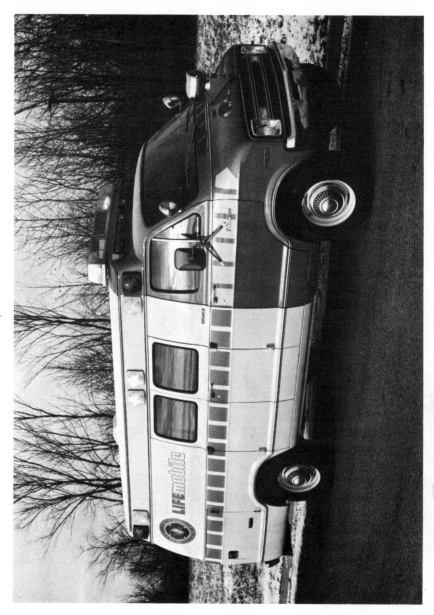

seven-foot long, eight-foot wide motor home could be converted to an emergency vehicle quite easily. It would have its own gas, water, and electricity and plenty of room for a team of medical personnel to treat several patients at once. He recommends that the community should pay for and operate the vehicle but it should be based at a general hospital.

Dr. Warm suggests that the size of the superambulance should not be a drawback. We are used to much larger fire engines which must rush to emergencies; the superambulance would be smaller than these.

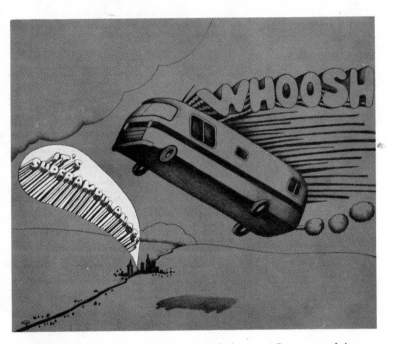

An artist's conception of the superambulance. (Courtesy of American Journal of Surgery)

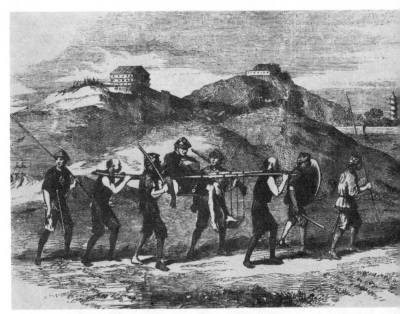

The Chinese developed a type of litter that made it possible to carry a wounded man in an upright sitting position, yet still support his legs as shown in the woodcut above. (Courtesy of Medical Tribune, *June 25, 1962)*

15

Ambulance Ideas from Around the World

Austria

All patients are transported on their side, never on their back, in the belief that this prevents pulmonary complications. All policemen and most doctors carry six units of plasma in their cars. All Viennese ambulances are over-equipped by U.S. standards. Each province in Austria has a fully stocked, one hundred-bed emergency hospital.

Belgium

There are two ambulance services—one operated by the government, the other by the Red Cross.

Canada

Canada provides health care to Eskimos in the Yukon and the Northwest Territory with medical airlift program, using helicopters and regular airplanes to bring patients to twelve hospitals and forty nursing stations.

England

HIGHLIGHTS OF LONDON AMBULANCE HISTORY

1879—Metropolitan Asylums Board provided a horse-drawn ambulance containing stretchers for two patients lying down and seats for attendants.

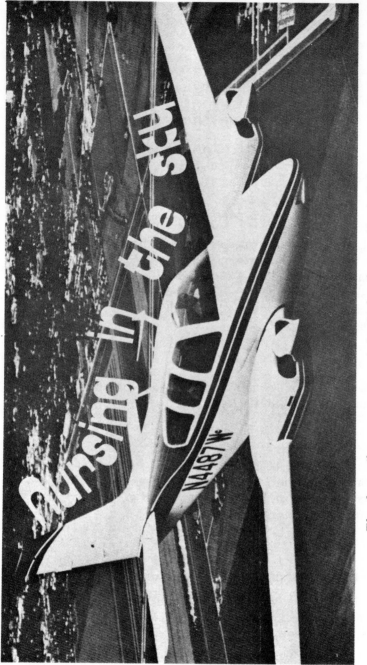

Nursing in the sky

The three pilot-nurse crews of the Saskatchewan Air Ambulance Service assure continuity of patient care for even the remotest community of the province. (Courtesy of The Canadian Nurse,

1882—London Horse Ambulance Service under presidency of the Duke of Cambridge. This service ended when the ambulances wore out.

1889—Mr. H. L. Bishoffscheim established his own service with sixty-two wheeled litters, operating from the police stations.

St. John Ambulance Association Service with thirty-five first aid stations in London, each having a wheeled litter and a stretcher.

1902—Steam ambulance used by Metropolitan Asylums Board, with eight stretchers, speeding five miles an hour.

1904—Motor Ambulance is first used.

River Ambulance Service was in use with three wharves and five steamers; however, this was discontinued in 1932.

1907—Electric motor ambulance service and fifty-two street call-boxes sponsored by the City Corporation came into use.

1915—Grand Duke Michael of Russia gave first motor-driven ambulance to the new London Ambulance Service.

LEEDS

In 1967 general practitioners set up a "road-accident aftercare" program to protect accident victims from being dragged from wrecks by well-meaning but unskilled helpers. Local police have the locations of doctors plotted on a map and dispatch the one closest to an accident. Since the program was initiated no one has died in transit.

In 1970, John H. Daykin, Chief Ambulance Officer in Leeds, commented that he knew of only two communities in the United Kingdom that had set up separate accident services within their ambulance service—Liverpool and London. Most ambulance services handled what is known as "sitting cases." In other words, the vehicles transport people from home to hospital out-patient treatment units. He said that emergency calls are quite unpredictable and if no ambulances are set aside for emergencies, the calls could come in when there are no conveyances available.

Ambulance design has improved greatly in the last several years. Each year the companies building ambulances add features to make the patient more comfortable with better means of treatment during transportation. Helicopters are also being improved as air ambulances. Stretchers and wheelchairs have become more sophisticated making it easier for the attendants as well as the patients. However, Dr. Daykin says, "Despite all the equipment improvement, none of it is any use unless the operators are trained to use the devices and can recognize the circumstances which calls for their use."

Ambulancemen are now required to have physical and mental examinations. They must also take an aptitude test and a driver's test in an ambulance. The *Millar Report,* Part I, a report by the Working Party on Ambulance Training and Equipment, made detailed recommendations on the method of training and the standard to be achieved. The National Joint Council for Manual Workers in Local Authority Services set up standards for pay and working conditions for ambulance attendants. The Department of Health and Social Security set up the Ambulance Services Advisory Committee which advises the Ministers of Health on Ambulance services.

The attitude toward ambulance services varies from those who are proud of them and spend a great deal for efficient services to those who begrudge any funds spent on good ambulance service.

The United Kingdom eventually hopes to be the best in the world in ambulance services. If all the nations would concentrate on this objective, think how many lives would be saved.

France, Paris

Necker Hospital has developed a shell mattress made of rubberized canvas and filled with small plastic granules. Then surrounded by air, it resembles a feather mattress and bulges up around the patient. Its developer says it could be of great value in transporting injured accident victims.

Germany

A stretcher bearer company was founded in Leipzig in 1703. The Jewish Hospital of Berlin, founded in the mid-eighteenth century, brought the sick person to the hospital on a stretcher.

Usually it was up to the patient or his family to get him to the hospital.

In the town of Halle in Germany an organized emergency transport system began about 1870. The development of heavy industries in the town precipitated more accidents which necessitated removal of victims by ambulance to places of treatment.

Rescuing companies formed throughout Germany in the 1870s to provide horse-drawn ambulances. The fire at the Vienna Theater in 1881 when four hundred people died, drew attention to the fact that first aid emergency plans were needed.

In 1885 the German Samariter Union developed all over Germany. The laborers in the heavy industries organized a trained staff to handle emergencies. By 1901, Halle had the first motorized ambulance vehicle in the city's history. The patient paid three marks for ambulance service. Merely having ambulances available did not solve the emergency problem. It was soon discovered that there must be trained attendants to ride the ambulances and treat the patient in transit. Halle had a direct train connection to Berlin and was an important industrial town.

Today, the German people have rotorized hospitals which will fly patients in emergencies. These flying operating rooms, developed in Germany, speed medical and surgical aid to any catastrophe site. A helicopter deposits the well-equipped gondola (Clinocopter) near the wounded and disembarks physicians and aids who open the gondola and begin to take care of the patients. The helicopter stands by to transport the patients to hospitals and, on return trips, can fly in additional supplies and personnel, as needed.

Special police ambulances for drunkards are employed in Hamburg, West Germany. They bring the drinkers to a special "sobering-up" station which has a doctor on call to screen medical emergencies.

Italy, Venice

The following article by Florence K. Lockerby, a contributing editor of *Hospitals* magazine describes ambulance service in Venice.

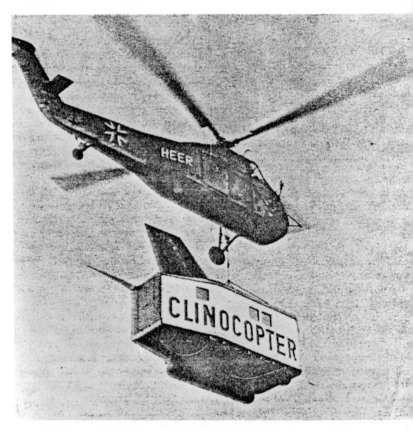

Flying operating room, developed in Germany. (Courtesy of Medical Tribune*)*

FLEET OF AMBULANCES EXPEDITES
EMERGENCY CARE IN VENICE *

BY

FLORENCE K. LOCKERBY

A twenty-four-hour transport and first-aid service provides emergency health care for all of the hospitals in and around the city

In order to expedite emergency health care for its 137,568 inhabitants and innumerable tourists, Venice, Italy, has solved its unique logistical problems by organizing and maintaining an aquatic ambulance service.

Built upon the mudbanks of the Venetian lagoon, this city of 100 islands is integrated by a network of canals and bridges to accommodate pedestrian traffic. Except for the piazzas (open squares), streets are less than four feet in width. Vaporettos (water busses), launches, small boats, and gondolas provide the only means of transportation throughout this canalized city.

Although Venice has no landbased vehicular traffic, which causes accidents in other cities, its narrow and slippery cobblestoned pavement and its canals can be hazardous. Pedestrians fall on the bridges, on the pavement, or into the canals.

For example, an American girl whom the ambulance staff attended was wearing clogs, and she slipped and fell on the damp pavement. Police called the Blue Cross (municipal ambulance service) station, and within 15 minutes, the ambulance docked at the site of the accident. The crew administered first aid, lifted the patient aboard the ambulance, and sped to Ospedele Civile in seven minutes. There the patient's fractured ankle was x-rayed and promptly and properly casted. If the accident had occurred during the winter, the ambulance attendants might have been forced to respond to the call on

*From Hospitals, J.A.H.A. *Reprinted with permission,* from Hospitals, Journal of the American Hospital Association, *50:48-50, 1976.*

foot and to carry the patient to the hospital in a litter, because the canal waters often rise so high that boats cannot clear the city's hundreds of small bridges.

In addition to the victims of orthopedic accidents, Blue Cross attends and transports patients who require hospitalization for other kinds of emergencies or for elective health care. Discharged patients also are transported by Blue Cross to their homes or to tourists' accommodations.

Ambulance personnel work in staggered shifts around the clock, seven days a week. Each of the five motorboat ambulances is equipped with first aid kits and with special litters that are fitted with back supports. (Cardio-pulmonary resuscitation equipment soon will be installed on each ambulance.) The well-trained crews are thoroughly familiar with the extensive and intricate canal system, and they speedily respond to emergency calls from the police, from hospitals, from first aid centers, and from private citizens. All Venetian hospitals maintain reserved docking space for the Blue Cross fleet.

The 2,000-bed Ospedele Civile, the largest of the five regional hospitals in the Veneto Region, includes 150 beds for patients admitted to the department of traumatology. The department's medical staff consists of seven physicians, who report that there is a high census of emergency admissions during the months from April through September, the peak of the tourist season. Tourists often mistrust Italian hospitals, and they insist on early discharge in order to return to their homelands and to their personal physicians. The physicians in the department of traumatology attribute this apprehension to the fact that the hospital buildings are very old.

In Italian public hospitals, the members of the medical staff are salaried. Medical care is included in the cost of hospitalization, which is covered by insurance. If a patient requests a better room, he must pay an additional amount for that accommodation and food service. In addition to public hospitals, there are many excellent private clinics in Italy. However, the rates for this kind of health care are prohibitively high.

The Netherlands, Amsterdam

The ambulances are all cream-colored, Dutch-built Chevrolets. Some use a swinging cot holder which permits placing a patient on a rack at the rear and swinging him smoothly into the ambulance.

Russia

Skoraya, the emergency medical care system in Russia, is set in motion by dialing 03. The ambulance then starts on its way to the emergency site. A physician, his assistant, and a nurse accompany the vehicle.

If the victim is under three years of age or has suffered a heart attack, poisoning, burns, shock, or neurological disorders, a specially equipped ambulance is dispatched along with a specially trained medical team.

The number of patients who die on the way to the Russian hospital is fantastically small. Dr. Patrick B. Storey of the University of Pennsylvania, who has studied the Soviet medical care system, believes that DOAs are rare because of the Soviet ability to get the patient to the hospital quickly with a fully capable medical team administering treatment in transit.

For twenty-four hours a day, Skoraya personnel, called feldshers, man the switchboard. The feldshers know where every ambulance is located at all times. They also have knowledge of each hospital's capability to handle emergencies. They have the means of dispatching ambulances and also direct them to the proper hospital facility. The Moscow Skoraya has some five hundred ambulances, one thousand physicians, and four thousand feldshers—for a city of approximately eight million people.

In the United States physicians once rode with ambulances to the scene of the emergency, but the practice has been discontinued. Instead, emergency technicians are being trained to ride the ambulances which are equipped with two-way telephone communication systems so that instructions may be transmitted from the physician to the technician if needed.

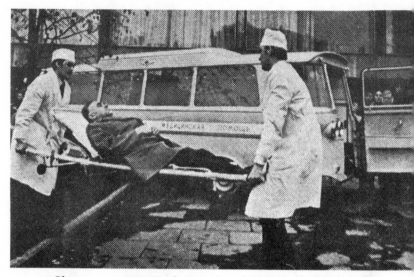

Skoraya team at work: Speed and skill make DOAs rare.

South Africa

The Air-Ambulance system has been in use in South Africa since the mid 1960s, but the Red Cross there needed a new and bigger aircraft. The Rotary Clubs of the area quickly raised funds to provide the new flying ambulance. Six volunteers acted as pilots (three of them were Rotarians) to fly "The Spirit of Rotary" on her missions of mercy.

These mobile medical squads can be located in high accident areas of South Africa. They are equipped with manual resuscitators, suction apparatus, first aid items, oxygen, heart monitoring equipment, etc. All calls are made with doctor on board who is experienced in accident injuries.

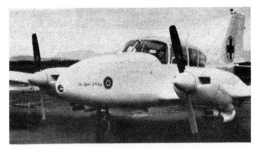

Air ambulance system.

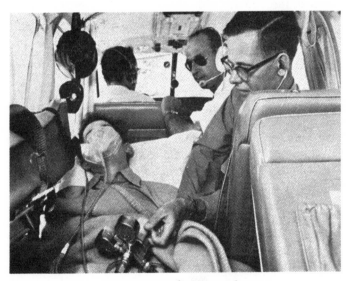

Mobile medical squad.

Sweden

Most emergency calls come in by people phoning "90.000"; in Malmo, a city of three hundred and fifty thousand people with one hospital containing several thousand beds, a second emergency number is used for calls requiring a doctor, a midwife, a chemist or a veterinarian.

16

An Ambulance Hobby

Dr. James W. Wengert, a psychiatrist in Omaha, Nebraska, has a very unusual hobby. He collects ambulances. Not full-sized ones, but miniatures. He has spent a great amount of time to locate specifications for building historical ambulances by searching through rare books and historical collections in libraries. When he finds the plans he is looking for, he sends the "specs" to craftsmen who build miniatures to scale.

When Dr. Wengert is not practicing psychiatry, he is doing the real thing at National Guard Camp with helicopter ambulances.

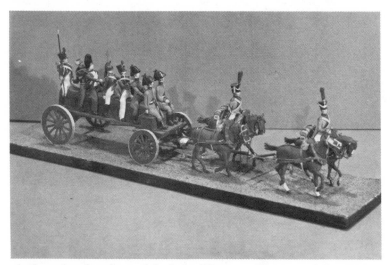

Antique handmade model of the "Sausage Wagon" of Dr. Percy, French army surgeon of the time of Napoleon and one of the earliest vehicles designed exclusively for a medical corps.

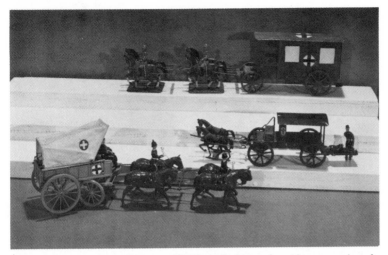

Top to bottom: *(1) German WWI ambulance by Algeyer uniquely camouflaged. (2) Ambulance by Heyde, Franco-Prussian War. (3) British ambulance of Queen Victoria's era by W. Britains.*

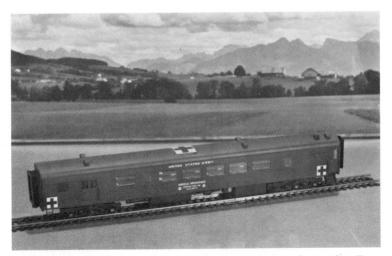

U.S. Army "rolling stocks" WWII used extensively in the Zone of Interior.

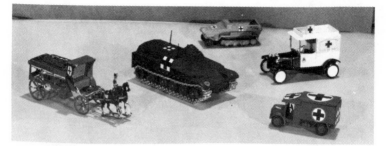

Left to Right: *(1) Toy manufacturers were quick to adopt the ambulance with markings very soon after the Red Cross was adopted. An early Italian model by Heyde. (2) The French still pioneer in ambulance design. A nuclear-chemical-biological warfare protected forward area ambulance AMX VCI by Solido. (3) Africa Corps half-track ambulance Sd. Kfz251/8. (4) Typically French, a 1920s Citroen ambulance of the Ville de Paris. (5) British Austin K2 ambulance in the colors of the 8th Army "Desert Rats."*

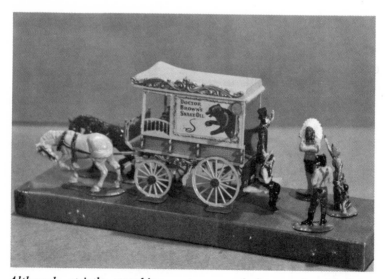

Although strictly speaking not an ambulance, the Medicine Wagon was a familiar sight in the early American West.

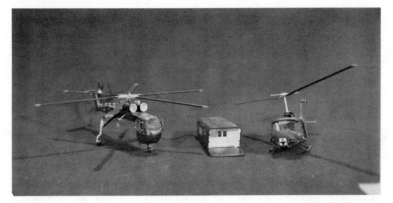

Helicopter ambulances starting in Korea and leading to whole squadrons in Vietnam of "Dustoff Units" have resulted in a dramatic improvement in battlefield to hospital life saving. Wounded in Vietnam were minutes away from full surgical facilities. Left to right: *(1) The Sikorsky Sky Crane can lift an entire surgical unit as a hospital ward in its pad. (2) The famous Vietnam "Huey." Whole squadrons of ambulance helicopters have been formed. The National Guard such as Nebraska's 24th Air Ambulance Company also has these units.*

17

Animal Ambulances

In 1902, Dr. W. H. Staniforth of Cleveland, Ohio, was the first veterinarian to have an automobile especially designed to transport sick and wounded animals to and from the hospital. The front portion of the ambulance was divided into two parts, the upper part was for cats, the lower for dogs. Each compartment was equipped with wire-covered ventilation slits and built-in water dishes.

In 1919, an ambulance for dogs appeared in London, England. It was the property of Animal's Hospital of London. The ambulance was drawn by a three horsepower motorcycle and looked like an ark. The ark was on springs, fitted with pneumatic tires and was padded inside.

England was the location for the first horse ambulance. The large truck ambulance had a revolving body. The inventor figured that horses like people, like to ride facing forward. The horse was loaded forward and for unloading the truck swung around on a pivot so that the horse could walk off frontwards. This eliminated the problems of backing the animal either way.

Today motor ambulances for animals are a naturally accepted part of this highly motorized era. Dr. J. F. Smithcors, who has compiled the information on animal ambulances and is the authority on the history of the veterinary practice, salutes those pioneers who led the way by adapting the latest mechanism to the needs of animals.

The following pictures come from Dr. J. F. Smithcor's private collection.

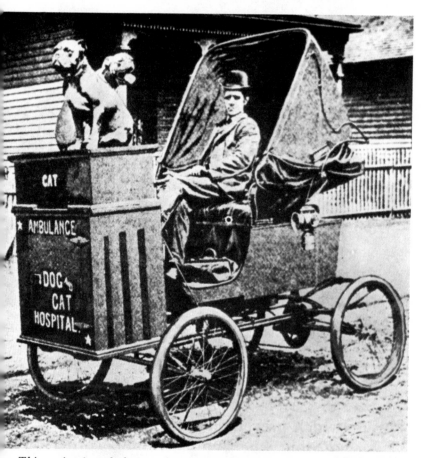

This animal ambulance, designed in 1902, was primarily used for the transport of dogs and cats. The front portion of the ambulance was divided into two parts; the upper part was for cats, the lower for dogs.

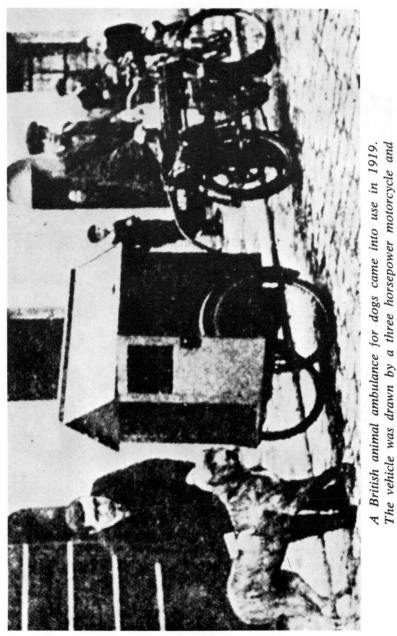

A British animal ambulance for dogs came into use in 1919. The vehicle was drawn by a three horsepower motorcycle and looked like an ark.

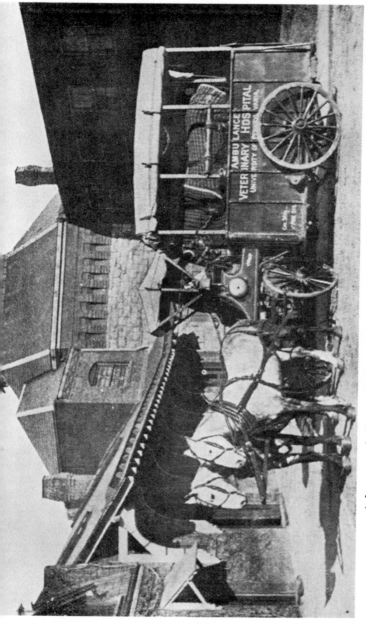

A horse ambulance of the University of Pennsylvania Veterinary Hospital, ca. 1890. Some of these ambulances were real show-pieces—painted fire-engine red with brass fittings. (Courtesy of University of Pennsylvania Bulletin)

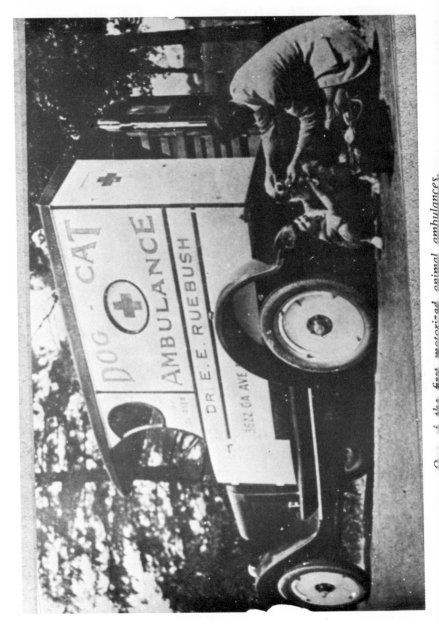

One of the first motorized animal ambulances.

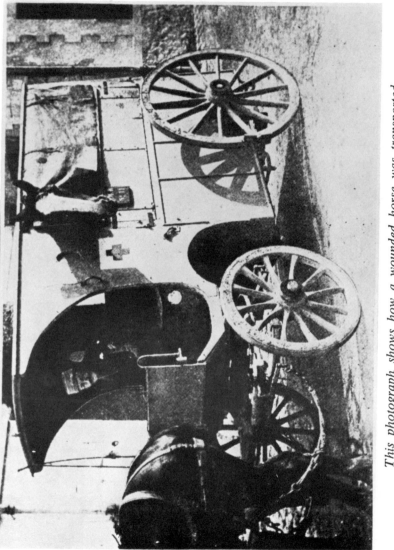

This photograph shows how a wounded horse was transported on the Marne front during the First World War.

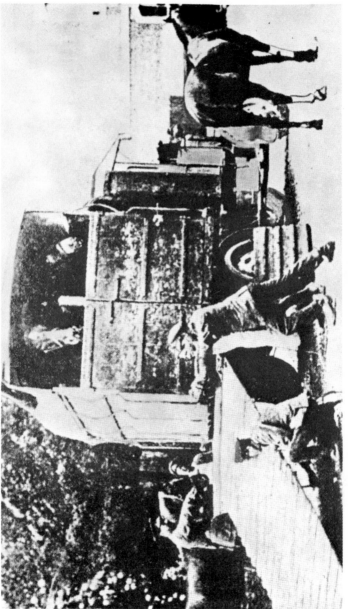

The first horse ambulance, designed in England, had a revolving body. The horse was loaded forward and for unloading the truck swung around on a pivot so that the horse could walk off frontwards. This method eliminated the problems of backing the animal either way.

Bibliography

Altman, L. K. "Science Academy Assails Nation's Emergency Care." *New York Times,* September 17, 1972.

"Ambulance Ideas from Other Countries." *Perspective* 6:9-10, 1971.

American Society of Anesthesiologists. "Community-wide Emergency Medical Services: Recommendations by the Committee on Acute Medicine of the American Society of Anesthesiologists." *Journal of the American Medical Association* 204: 595-602, 1968.

Arp, L. J., et al, "An Emergency Air-ground Transport System for Newborn Infants with Respiratory Distress." *Pennsylvania Medicine* 72:74-76, 1969.

Artz, Curtis P. "Presidential Address: Make Your Commitment." *Journal of Trauma* 12:99-103, 1972.

Ash, R. V. "Transport of Sick and Wounded in Uncivilized Countries, Bearing Especially on the Late Kaffir Campaigns." *Transactions of the International Medical Congress* 2:501-504, 1881.

Baker, George L. "Design and Operation of a Van for the Transport of Sick Infants." *American Journal of Diseases of Children* 18:743, 1969.

————. "Special Van Gives Babies Start on Survival." *Journal of the American Medical Association* 209:1826, 1969.

Barnes, Joseph K. "The Medical and Surgical History of the War of Rebellion (1861-1865)." Washington, D.C.: Government Printing Office, 1870.

Barnsley, R. E. "A Search Rewarded—Discovery of Horse Drawn Ambulance Wagon." *Lancet* 2:1372, 1958.

Barton, Clara. *The Red Cross.* Washington, D.C.: American National Red Cross, 1898.

Beatty, W. K. and Marks, G. *Women in White.* New York: Scribner's Sons, 1972.

Boyd, D. R.; Flashner, B. A.; Nyhus, L. M. and Phillips, C. W. "Clinical and Epidemiologic Characteristics of Non-surviving Trauma Victims in an Urban Environment." *Journal of the National Medical Association* 64:1-7, 1972.

Brooks, Stewart. *Civil War Medicine.* Springfield, Illinois: Charles C. Thomas, 1966.

Brown, R. "Camel Stretcher Carrier: Method of Carrying Casualties on a Stretcher—For Use with Camels." *Royal Army Medical Corps. Journal.* 71:48-9, 1938.

"Buck Ambulance Celebrates Six Decades of Service to Community." *AID, Journal of the Ambulance Association of America.* March 1973, p. 5.

Carlisle, R. J. "An Account of Bellevue Hospital—1893." New York: New York Society of the Alumni of Bellevue Hospital.

"Centenary of Solferino." *New England Journal of Medicine* 260: 1343, 1959.

Clarke, J. T. "Canada's First Ambulance Train." *Military Surgery* 68: 649-50, 1931.

Clements, B. A. "Memoirs of Jonathan Letterman, 1883." *Journal Military Service Institute,* September 1883.

Collins, Herbert R. *Red Cross Ambulance of 1898 in the Museum of History and Technology.* Contributions from the Museum of History and Technology, Paper 50, Bulletin 241. Smithsonian Institute, 1965.

Commission on Emergency Medical Services, American Medical Association. *Accidental Death and Disability: The Neglected Disease of Modern Society.* Washington, D.C.: National Academy of Sciences National Research Council.

————. "Developing Emergency Medical Services—Guidelines for Community Councils." Chicago: American Medical Association.

Davy, R. "On Invalid Transit." *British Medical Journal* 2:1142, 1882.

————. "Remarks on the Transit of Invalids." *British Medical Journal* 2:553, 1876.

Daykin, J. H. "The Development of Ambulance Services in the United Kingdom." *Royal Society of Health Journal* 90:5, 1970.

Delafield, R. *Report on the Art of War in Europe: 1854, 1855, 1856*. Washington: George W. Bowman, 1861.

Dible, J. H. *Napoleon's Surgeon*. London: William Heinemann Medical Books, Ltd., 1970.

"Digest of Surveys Conducted 1965 to March 1971—Ambulance Services and Hospital Emergency Departments." USPHS, Division of Emergency Health Services.

"Directory of Emergency Physicians." *Medical Opinion* 1:29, August, 1972.

Drum, W. F. "Ambulance Train in 1864." *Military Surgery* 70: 607-611, 1932.

Edwards, A. G. "Helicopter Rescue Service." *Lancet* 1:470-72, 1958.

Ellis, C. *Military Transport of World War I*. New York: Macmillan Company, 1970.

————. *Military Transport of World War II*. New York: Macmillan Company, 1971.

"Emergency Medicine: Emerging Specialty." *Medical Digest* 16:79-82, September 1972.

Emily Dunning Barringer: Bowery to Bellevue, the Story of New York's First Woman Ambulance Surgeon. New York: W. W. Norton and Company, 1950.

Evans, J. "Motor Barge as Ambulance Ship." *British Medical Journal* 2:59-60, 1941.

Farrington, J. D. "Transportation of the Injured." *Postgraduate Medicine* 48:139-43, 1970.

Fletcher, N. Corbet. *Saint John Ambulance Association: Its History and Its Part in the Ambulance Movement*. Saint John's Gate: Saint John's Ambulance Association, 1930.

Gearty, G. F., et al, "Pre-hospital Coronary Care Services." *British Medical Journal* 3:33, 1971.

"Geisinger Medical Center Becomes Disaster Headquarters in

Danville, Pennsylvania Flood." *Group Practice,* July 1972, p. 19-26.

Grace, W. J. "The Mobile Coronary Care Unit and the Intermediate Coronary Care Unit in the Total Systems Approach to Coronary Care." *Chest* 58:363-68, 1970.

_____and Chadbourn, J. A. "The Mobile Coronary Care Unit." *Chest* 55:425, 1969.

Graf, W. S. "Problems in Establishing a Mobile Coronary Unit." *Medical Opinion & Review,* December 1970, p. 72-78.

Green, Ora M. "Horse Ambulance." *RN* 19:73, September 1956.

Gutowski, Walter. "First Aid Afloat." *Safety Maintenance* 121: 43, February 1961.

Hampton, Oscar P. "The Committee on Trauma of the American College of Surgeons—1922-1972." *American College of Surgeons. Bulletin.* June 1972, p. 7-13.

Henderson, P. H. "Ambulance Transport in Undeveloped Countries." *Royal Society of Medicine. Proceedings.* 24:35-51, 1931.

Hess & Eisenhardt. "A History of Achievement Since 1876." *Cincinnati Magazine,* June 1968.

Hoffman, C. A. "Emergencies Speak the Same Language." *Medical Opinion,* December 1972, p. 51-54.

Holloway, Ronald M. "New York City's Experience in Improving Ambulance Service." *Health Services Reports* 87:446-40, 1972.

Holmes, Mara. "Survival by the Numbers—Emergency Medicine Plan like Russia's Could Save U.S. Lives." *National Observer,*

Horner, W. E. "Ambulance." *American Cyclopedia of Practice of Medicine* 1:338-41, 1834.

Hornung, C. P. *Wheels Across America.* New York: Dover Press, 1959.

Hulme, Fred. "Fore . . . Make Way for a Golf Course Rescue Vehicle." *National Observer,* September 15, 1973, p. 9.

Hume, Edgar Erskine. *Medical Work of the Knights Hospitallers of Saint John of Jerusalem.* Baltimore: Johns Hopkins Press, 1940.

Huntley, Henry C. "Emergency Care System for National Political

Conventions in Miami Beach, Florida." *Medical Opinion,* August 1972, p. 20.

———— "Emergency Health Services for the Nation." *Public Health Reports* 85:517, 1970.

———— "How Is Emergency Care in Your Community?" *Emergency Medicine,* April 1972, p. 51-55.

Isler, Charlotte. "Dial 911 for the Coronary Ambulance." *RN* 32:48-51, August 1969.

"Jonathan Letterman: Father of American Military Ambulance Service." *Clinical Medicine* 49:153-54, 1942.

Joynson, William. "Horse-ambulances in Connection with Hospitals." *British Medical Journal* 1:909-910, 1885.

Kaiser, W., Piechocki, W. and Suhs, H. "Del Anfange Eines Organisierten Krankentransports am Beispel der Stadt." *Geschichte der Medizin.*

Kane, Joseph N. *Famous First Facts.* Third edition. New York: H. W. Wilson Co., 1964.

Keggi, K. J. "Yale Confronts Urban Trauma." *Roche Medical Image and Commentary.*

Kennedy, Robert H. "Ambulances are More than Vehicles." *Journal of Trauma* 3:393, 1963.

Kirschner, M. "Surgical Ambulance with Roentgen Service, Operating Room and Car for Seriously Wounded, for Use During Campaign and in Time of Public Calamities." *Chirurg* 10:713-17, 1938.

Knapp, J. "Carriage for Cholera Patients." *London Medical Gazette,* 1882, p. 825.

Lemcke, J. A. "The *Fanny Bullitt* and the Civil War." *S & D Reflector* 7:21-27. Published by Sons & Daughters of Pioneer Rivermen, June 1970.

Lewis, Richard P. "A Town that Does: Columbus, Ohio, Mobile Coronary Care Unit," *Emergency Medicine* 3:57, July 1971.

Little, Keith. "Profile of an Accident Flying Squad." *British Medical Journal* 3:807-810, September 30, 1972.

"Lives Saved vs. Dollars Spent Transporting Emergency Patients." *Perspective* 6:9-17, 1971.

Lockerby, Florence. "Fleet of Ambulances Expedites Emergency Care in Venice." *Hospitals* 50:48-50, 1976.

Longmore, Thomas. *A Treatise on the Transport of Sick and Wounded Troops.* London: Her Majesty's Stationery Office, 1869.

McKenny, Ellen M. "History of the Motorized Ambulance Transport." *Military Medicine* 132:819-22, 1967.

Marten, E. T. "Modern Ambulances Have Developed from Rude Beginnings." *Modern Hospital* 42:43-46, 1934.

Medical Requirements for Ambulance Design and Equipment. Washington, D.C.: National Academy of Sciences National Research Council Task Force, September, 1968.

Medical World News Staff. "The Crisis in Emergency Care." *Medical World News* December 4, 1970; April 16, 1970.

Mennear-Dubas, Susan. "Sea Rescue." *Family Health* 9:40-43, 1977.

Miles, A. B. "The Charity Hospital Ambulance Services, New Orleans, Louisiana." *New Orleans Medical & Surgical Journal* 13:51-56, 1885.

"Military and Naval Medicine Mechanics in Medicine: The Military Ambulance." *British Journal Clinical Practice* 14:154, 1960.

Military Medical Manual. Fourth edition. Harrisburg, Pennsylvania: The Military Service Publishing Co.

"Minimal Equipment for Ambulances—American College of Surgeons Committee on Trauma." American College of Surgeons. Bulletin 52:92-96, 1967.

"Modified Coronary Ambulance." *Medical Journal of Australia* 2:1182, 1969.

Murphy, Stephen P. "San Diego Plan for Emergency Services." *American Journal of Nursing.* 72:1615-19, 1972.

Nagel, Eugene L. and Hirschman, J. "Pre-hospital Care: Time for Decision." *Medical Opinion* 7:28, December, 1971.

Newhouse, N. H. "Alligator Ambulance." *U. S. Navy Medical Bulletin* 40:719-20, 1942.

Noble, Iris. *First Woman Ambulance Surgeon—Emily Barringer.* New York: Julian Messner, 1962.

Oertel, Mary R. "Training Emergency Medical Technicians in New Mexico." *Health Services Reports* 87:195-99, 1972.

Otis, George A. *Report to the Surgeon General on the Transport of Sick and Wounded by Pack Animals.* War Department Surgeon General's Office Circular Number 9, March 1, 1877. Reprint by Sol Lewis, 1974.

Packard, Francis R. *History of Medicine in the United States* Vol. 1. New York: Hafner Publishing Co., 1963.

Pantridge, J. F. and Geddes, J. S. "A Mobile Intensive Care Unit in the Management of Myocardial Infarction." *Lancet* 2:271-73, 1967.

"Port of London Health Craft." *Royal Society of Health Journal* 82:228, 1962.

"Portraits of the Past—Dr. Isadore Faust, Intern on Ambulance Duty." *Bronx-Lebanon Hospital Center Newsletter.* Bronx, New York.

Poynter, F. N. L. *Medicine and Surgery in the Great War (1914-1918).* Exhibition Catalogue #4. London: Wellcome Institute of the History of Medicine, 1968.

Preston, Robert H. "Hospital Transports with Special Reference to the Steamboat *Allen Collier* and the Cincinnati Branch of the U.S. Sanitary Commission." *Ohio State Medical Journal* 53:1037-38, 1957.

Rideing, W. H. "Hospital Life in New York." *Harper's New Monthly Magazine* 57:171-89, 1878.

Roberts, Stuart, et al. "Medicopter: An Airborn Intensive Care Unit." *Annals of Surgery* 172:325, September 1970.

"Rotary Purchase of Airplane Ambulance for South African Red Cross—1971." *Rotarian,* October 1972.

"Rotarized Hospital Flies to Patients." *Medical Tribune* #26, June 25, 1962.

Safar, Peter. "Ambulance Design and Equipment for Mobile Intensive Care." *Archives of Surgery* 102:163-71, 1971.

————. "Community Concern Sparks Ambulance Service." *Modern Hospital* 13:93-98, 1969.

————. "Emergency Medical Technicians as Allied Health Professionals. Anesthesia and Analgesia." *Current Researchers* 51:27-34, 1972.

――――― and Brose, R. A. "Ambulance Design and Equipment for Resuscitation." *Archives of Surgery* 90:343-48, 1965.

Schindele, Ernst F. "First Ambulance Boat Starts Free Medical Service on Long Island Sound." (Press release and Personal Correspondence.) 1976.

Schwartz, Mortimer. "Mobile Coronary Care Unit." *Medical Opinion & Review* 6:52, 1970.

Scientific American 75:284, October 10, 1896. Velocipede.

Scientific American 82:148, 1900. Electric Automobile.

Scientific American 108:316, April 5, 1913. Streetcar Ambulance.

Scott, T. E. "New Pack Saddle Litter for Panama Jungle." *Military Surgery* 79:203-207, 1936.

Sewall, C. A. "A New Extemporaneous Litter, Copied After the Mojave Indian Method of Carrying the Wounded." *Medical Record* 38:461, 1890.

Shepard, K. S. "Air Transportation of High Risk Infants Utilizing a Flying Intensive Care Nursery." *Journal of Pediatrics* 77:148, 1970.

Simpson, R. K. "Airplane Ambulance: Its Use in War." *Military Surgery* 64:35-48, 1929.

Skinner, Henry Alan. *The Origin of Medical Terms*. Baltimore: Williams & Wilkins, 1949.

Smellie, Hugh M. "An Ambulance Chair." *British Medical Journal* 1:1133, 1891.

Smith, J. T. "Review of Life and Work of Jonathan Letterman." *Johns Hopkins Hospital Bulletin,* August 1916.

Smith, Rhea Marsh. *Spain, A Modern History*. Ann Abor, Michigan: University of Michigan Press, 1965.

Smithcors, J. F. *The Veterinarian in America,* 1625-1975. Santa Barbara, California: American Veterinary Publications, Inc., 1975.

Snook, Roger. "Accident Flying Squad." *British Medical Journal* 2:569-78, 1972.

Talbott, John H. *A Biographical History of Medicine*. New York: Grune & Stratton, 1970.

"Training of Ambulance Personnel and Others Responsible for Emergency Care of the Sick and Injured at the Scene and During Transport." Washington, D.C.: Superintendent of Documents.

Tunis, Edwin. *Wheels, A Pictorial History.* New York: World Publishing Co., 1955.

Uhley, Herman. "Ambulance Hot Line for Coronary Care." *Roche Medical Image and Commentary* 1971.

———— "Electrocardiographic Telemetry From Ambulances. A Practical Approach to Mobile Coronary Units." *American Heart Journal* 80:838, December 1970.

Warm, H. "Tomorrow's Ambulance: An Emergency Room on Wheels." *American Journal of Surgery* 120:780, December, 1970.

Warren, James V. "Mobile Coronary Care in the Logistics of Surviving a Heart Attack." *Medical Opinion & Review* 6:14, November 1970.

Waters, John M. "A Synopsis of Emergency Medical Services for a Large City." *Journal of Trauma* 12:95-6, January 1972.

Wangenstein, O. H., and Wangenstein, S. D. "Successful Pre-Listerian Management of Compound Fractures—Crowther, Larrey and Bennion." *Surgery* 69:811-24, 1971.

Webb, Kenneth M. "Private Foundations Meet the Problem." *Medical Opinion,* March 1973.

Whiteman, Maxwell. *Mankind and Medicine.* Philadelphia: Einstein Medical Center, 1966.